S.C.H.O.O.L.
Yourself
into Shape

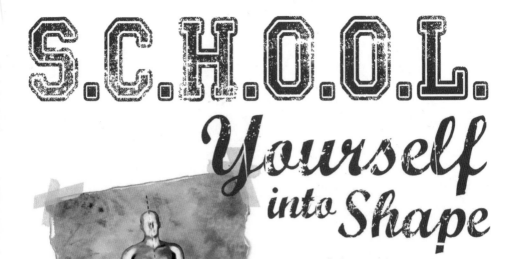

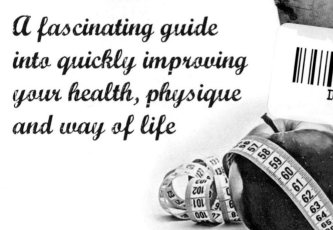

A fascinating guide into quickly improving your health, physique and way of life

D1446562

By Kevin Bruce White

Table of Contents

Introduction

So I guess this is my introduction, the part of the book where I answer the unheard question, why did you write this book? Perhaps the better question is…Why are you reading this book? At any rate, we'll revisit why you're reading this book later. However for now, I'll give you a few of the endless reasons I started typing out my thoughts and advice. I'd like to think it was the annoying but comical phrases that constantly regurgitated from clients and friends alike. I'm sure you've heard them, or possibly spewed them out yourself.

"Kevin, I've been exercising every day and I'm still not losing weight." This coming out the mouths of people who had worked out for a whopping three days! Oh and here is another one that I heard close to a million times.

"How come my friend eats junk food all the time and looks awesome?" To which I would reply, "Well, a hummingbirds metabolism is so fast, it can eat up to three times it's bodyweight in one day. Do you also compare yourself to a hummingbird? Stop comparing yourself to others and focus on yourself"

Okay one more and then I'll get back to the introduction, I promise.

"Kevin, I need to lose 25 pounds in 2 weeks for this wedding, can you help me?" There was always a few seconds of silence following this verbal madness, usually accompanied with a bizarre look upon my face, and finally there was my response "I am not a magician, nor have I ever performed magic in my life. So please tell me why you're asking a personal trainer to perform magic?

That's just a small fraction of what I heard every day over the last 25 years, and rightfully so because I was a personal trainer and fitness consultant. I took in the questions, and answered them always, even with an occasional eye roll. With that being said, no matter how taxing it became hearing those questions time and again, it was far outshined by the joy I received witnessing friends, clients, and colleagues revitalize their lives by improving their fitness. On the other hand, nothing frustrated me more than watching people who were either misdirected or not self-accountable fail repeatedly trying to get in shape. This followed by the dreaded…"I might as well give up I'm never going to get in shape." I guess ultimately it was witnessing people go through that feeling of being defeated that made me think, "I'm going to write a book that gives the reader a prescription for getting in shape and preserving it"

Introduction

This book will teach you the S.C.H.O.O.L. approach to better fitness. It's my formula for remembering the key components needed to quickly get in shape, and preserving it. The acronym S.C.H.O.O.L represents structure, consistency, habits, overcoming obstacles, and lifestyle. This approach eliminates the over thinking involved in trying to get in shape, and replaces it with clarity. You will come to realize that there is a reason they're called fad diets and workouts, and in most cases they produce temporary results, regardless of who has endorsed them. In addition, you'll learn that it takes less than 2000 hours to get in shape and revitalize your spirit. That's right 2000 hours! That equates to 83 days, or about twelve weeks to revive your body, mind, and way of life. Moreover, you'll become conscious of how easy it is to stay fit forever.

So take a stroll over to the nearest mirror, look at yourself, and think of every possible reason why you want to improve your health, figure, and lifestyle. I don't care if you think some of the reasons might be stupid, pointless, or even absurd, go write them down. If they came to mind while you were standing in front of that mirror, then to you, they must have some type of significance. Then write down all the things that you are accountable for in your life. Think hard, maybe it's your spouse, children, job, or school. Once you've done that, find the consequences that you avoid by remaining accountable to these particulars. For example, not committing to your job could lead to unemployment, and not committing to your partner might lead to the single life. It's these types of repercussions that raise awareness and accountability, and remind us that we might ultimately have to answer to our boss or partners. However, when it comes to being self-accountable for improving our fitness, so many of us fail because there is no one to answer to, except ourselves. Remember that you only have one body, and if you don't take care of it, it will not take care of you. Also realize, if you don't have your health, you don't have anything. Make a pledge to yourself, make yourself accountable, read every chapter of this book, and reap the benefits of a new you!

Onto Chapter One!

CHAPTER
one
STRUCTURE

During the introduction I mentioned a formula that I came up with called S.C.H.O.O.L.

Structure, Consistency, Habits, Overcoming Obstacles, and Lifestyle

This acronym is a tool to remind you of the important factors needed to get and stay in shape. I've dedicated each chapter of this book to one of the components above. In this chapter I'll discuss how important structure is, and how the lack of it can destroy your entire game plan.

I'm sure you've heard of many diet plans and weight loss programs, and I'm sure several of you have tried them with no success. Perhaps some of you tried them, got results, but in time went right back to where you started. I'm not going to sit here and bash these programs because a lot of them have produced great results for the people who have tried them. Take the P90X programs, many people have had a tremendous amount of success with these programs, and there's a reason. Not only is the program good, but it's a program that creates structure for the user. Yes, the workouts are great, and there is a variety of cross training involved. However, for 90 days you've got everything laid out in front of you, and all you have to do is follow it, no thinking involved. The program consists of a nutrition guide, fitness plan, calendar, and series of DVDs demonstrating a variety of techniques. Just push "play" follow the workout and nutrition guide, and "Bam" 90 days later you've made some improvements. On the other hand, what happens after 90 days? This is where so many people fall apart. You bust your ass, follow a program, start feeling better, lose some weight, and then somewhere along the way you become lost.

Somehow your motivation starts to disappear, or you become more and more distracted.

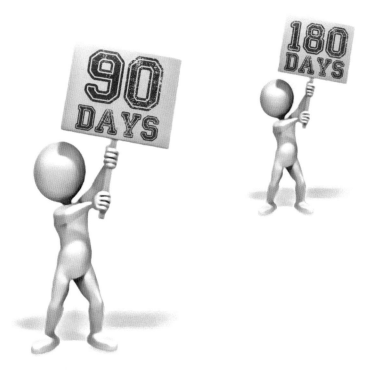

Then eventually you relinquish your structure completely and it's over. Sound familiar? Well, you're going to learn how to take that structure beyond 90 days, and make it a permanent addition to your life. One of the first things you need to know about structure is…it's your structure. Everyone's structure is different, and trying to lay out your game plan the way someone else does, could set you up for failure. You have to find your happy mediums with exercise, nutrition, and sleep. Following someone else's exercise plan or diet because they look awesome, or they just recently lost a bunch of weight, is a quick way to disappointment. Let's start with your diet, because nutrition is the most important part on the road to getting in shape.

DIET

Imagine your metabolism as a fire, and if you ate a small healthy meal that would be like adding a log to that fire. In contrast, eating a shitty meal or over eating is like dousing that fire with water, and not eating any meals is like letting the fire burn out. Don't you want your metabolism, that fire inside you, burning strong? The traditional way of eating has always been three meals, breakfast, lunch, and dinner. However, many experts claim that eating five to six smaller meals throughout the day was more effective when trying to lose weight and keep it off. There is no scientific proof that eating small meals, more often throughout the day boosts your metabolism, but I do favor this approach. It has always worked with my schedule, and I'll emphasize MY schedule. When I follow this approach, hunger usually isn't an issue, the multiple meals help regulate my blood sugar and control my cravings. More importantly, it helps me build and spare muscle, and the amount of muscle you have does determine the overall speed of your resting metabolism. Nonetheless, some people who experiment with five to six meals a day find themselves struggling trying to take in smaller portions at each meal. Also many people encounter problems making time to plan and prepare for all of those healthy meals. This is where you have to recognize what approach is best for you, screw what everyone else is doing, and that includes me. You need to figure out what's more achievable for you... three, four, five, or six meals. Just remember you have to eat multiple healthy meals throughout the day. Once you've done that, the next step is to figure out what your current caloric intake is, followed by finding the ideal caloric intake for yourself. In most cases, you need to reduce your caloric intake to lose weight. However, sometimes it just involves changing the type of calories you're eating. The illustration below gives you an example of eating roughly 2000 calories per day by way of three, four, five, and six meals a day.

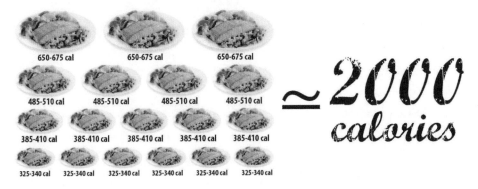

If your diet consists of bacon and cake, then 2000 calories is not a lot of food, and you'll have to really focus over the next few paragraphs.

Realizing what are good calories and bad calories is huge. Whole foods are examples of good calories, and by whole foods I mean foods that are in their natural non-processed state. Foods such as fruits, vegetables, yogurt, milk, eggs, seafood (preferably wild), pork, beef, chicken, nuts, seeds, water, honey, and juices in moderation. Just remember foods that have one ingredient are a plus. In contrast, processed, fried, wheat based, and genetically modified foods are bad calories.

Now just because a certain food falls under the good calorie group, that does not give you the green light to plow down 5 pounds of beef, and top it off with 4 cups of yogurt smothered with honey. If you take this route, you'll exhaust your daily calories by the end of your first meal. The key is to choose wisely, and to portion control. Learn about the foods you consume, and how many calories they have. Also learn the nutritional facts on the foods you take in. Find out how much protein, carbohydrates, and fats they contain. Educating yourself is a huge tool, and it's one of the reasons you're reading this book.

Next, you need to understand how to put together a healthy well-balanced meal. In the introduction I mentioned fad diets and how they produce temporary results. This is because they confuse the hell out of people. Low-carb/high-protein, no-carb/high-protein, high-carb/low-fat, Atkins, cabbage soup diet, and the HCG diet to name a few. WTF, trying to choose a fad diet will have your eyes spinning around in your head like a broken slot machine. How can you figure out which method to choose from when so many are out there, and they all seem to negate each other. This I do know, there are six essential nutrients, and essential nutrients must be provided by food. These nutrients are necessary for the body to function properly, and these six essential nutrients include carbohydrates, protein, fat, vitamins, minerals and water. If you're on a diet, or your daily food intake lacks one or more of these nutrients, you're just opening the door for disease.

Carbohydrates are the main energy source for the brain. Without carbohydrates, the body could not function properly. **Fats** store energy, insulate us and protect our vital organs. Fats also act as messengers, helping proteins do their jobs. **Proteins** do most of the work in cells and are they are also required for the structure, function, and regulation of the body's tissues and organs. **Minerals** support the growth of strong teeth and bones, nerve function, blood clotting and muscle contraction. They also help in cell repair, regulating body temperature, conversion of food into energy and in the breakdown of fat, proteins and carbohydrates.

Vitamins produce energy, protect cells from damage, guide mineral utilization, and regulate cell and tissue growth. Water helps to maintain homeostasis in the body and transports nutrients to cells. **Water** also assists in removing waste products from the body. These are just a few examples of the functions each of these nutrients are responsible for in our bodies.

Bottom line, these nutrients have important functions, and they work alongside of each other. I understand that preparing a meal with all the essential nutrients will not always come as a convenience. Many of us have time constraints as well as other obstacles, and that's why we will address these concerns in later chapters. In the meantime, I want you to think about the following when you're preparing your meals. The necessary nutrients that you should have at every meal are carbohydrates, fats, proteins, and water, and these are macronutrients. Vitamins and minerals are micronutrients and they're found in all the foods we consume.

MICRONUTRIENTS
- Vitamins
- Minerals

MACRONUTRIENTS
- Water
- Carbohydrates
- Proteins
- Lipids (fats)

Okay readers this is where you're really going to have to bear with me a little. Sometimes trying to learn about nutrients, ratios, and formulas can really feel like school. Remember, the name of the book is "School Yourself into Shape." With that being said, learning this is very important, and there are far more boring things in this world. For example, imagine being a kangaroo on a trampoline. So deal with it!

Just a quick reminder, macronutrients are nutrients containing calories that supply us with energy, and they consist of proteins, carbohydrates, and fats. The calories in each gram of macronutrients are as follows:

Proteins - Contains 4 calories per gram

Fats - Contain 9 calories per gram

Carbohydrates - Contains 4 calories per gram

Now that you understand what nutrients need to be included in your meals, and how many calories are in a gram of each of these nutrients (proteins, fats, and carbohydrates). Now, we need to find a good macronutrient ratio.

Your macronutrient ratio is the percentage of carbs, protein, and fat that you eat.

Most nutritional organizations suggest that your calories be made up of 55-65% carbohydrates, 10-15% protein, and 20-25% fat. This is also the ratio that I feel everyone should at least start out with.

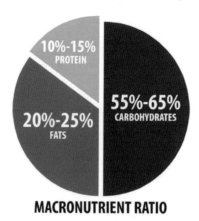

MACRONUTRIENT RATIO

So you're asking, "How do I count my macronutrients, and how do I know I'm taking in the recommended percentage?" Once you've determined how many calories you will be eating per day, then you can determine the macronutrient makeup of your diet.

For example let's use a 2000 calorie per day diet, with a macronutrient ratio consisting of 25 percent fat, 15 percent protein, and 60 percent carbohydrates.

First, we need to calculate the number of calories that you should get from fats, protein, and carbohydrates each day. If your diet allows 2,000 calories per day, with 25 percent of your calories coming from fat. You need to take the percentage of fat and multiply it by your daily caloric intake (0.25 x 2,000 = 500), which equals 500 calories per day from fat. Similarly, you'll get 0.15 x 2,000 = 300 calories from protein each day, and finally your carbohydrate requirement which is 0.60 x 2,000 = 1200 calories per day.

Second, figure out how many grams of fat, protein, and carbohydrates you're allowed each day. If each gram of fat has 9 calories and your daily fat allowance is 500 calories. You need to take your daily calories of fat which would be 500, and divide it by 9 the amount of calories that are in a gram of fat (500/9 =55.5), which equals 55.5 grams of fat each day. Likewise, each gram of protein has 4 calories and your daily protein allowance is 300 calories. Therefore, 300/4 = 75 grams of protein each day. Finally, each gram of carbohydrates has 4 calories and your daily allowance is 1200 calories. Therefore, 1200/4 = 300 grams of carbohydrates each day.

For all of you that suck at math, there is this thing called a calculator, it's amazing. Using the formula above can help you easily find how many grams of each macronutrient you need per day to support the ratio you've chosen. So if you were eating three meals a day you would be taking in about 18 grams of fat per meal (55/3=18), 25 grams of protein per meal (75/3 = 25), and 100 grams of carbohydrates at each meal (300/3 = 100). On the other hand, if you were eating 6 meals a day you would be taking in about 9 grams of fat per meal (55/6 = 9), 12.5 grams of protein per day (75/6 = 12.5), and 50 grams of carbohydrates at each meal (300/6 = 50).

In time you'll learn to experiment with your macronutrient ratios, and you'll realize that you'll have to adjust the ratios based on what you're trying to accomplish or what type of activities you're doing. If you're trying to lose more fat, then you might want to bring up your protein and fat ratios and lower your carbohydrate ratio. If you're doing endurance sports you might want to raise your carbohydrate and fat ratios, and lower your protein ratio. The important thing is to learn what works for your body, and to always include at least some portion of all the macronutrients.

A few more important factors to consider are *maintaining long satiation after meals*. Satiation is the feeling or condition of being full after eating food. Fat and proteins trigger satiation for longer periods than carbohydrates do, so diets that are very high in carbohydrates will probably have you feeling hungry between meals. So having a macronutrient ratio that is very high in carbohydrates could lead to cravings between meals, especially if you're only eating three or four meals a day. If you're going to eat a fewer larger meals, as opposed to many smaller meals throughout the day, then you might want to consider slightly bringing up your protein and fat ratios to prevent feeling hungry between meals.

In the same breath avoid lowering your carbohydrate to minimal or non-existence levels. This is very common among many fad diets, because it's a quick way to lose weight. Nevertheless, the results are short-lived, and people quickly discover it's hard to continue taking in such a limited amount of carbohydrates over an extended time. In addition, if your carbohydrate ratio is that low, then naturally your protein and fat ratios are very high. Diets that are too high in protein can lead to constipation, bad breath, and severe lethargy. Long-term high protein diets have also been linked to kidney problems, osteoporosis, colon cancer and heart disease. This is why most nutritional organizations suggest somewhere around 55-65% carbohydrates, 10-15% protein, and 20-25% fat.

Remember, the ratios are far less important when viewed in the context of what you're actually putting in your body. Think fruits and vegetables for good carbohydrates. You can't make a poor fruit or vegetable choice. They all contain vitamins, minerals and phytonutrients, not to mention some our considered super foods because of their high antioxidant levels. A good protein source is grass-fed meats, dairy and wild fish. Grass-fed meats might put a little dent in your wallet, but they are free of hormones, antibiotics and other chemicals. Avoid farm raised fish if possible, wild fish is usually not injected with chemicals, and all the other bullshit. Organic dairy and eggs from free-range chickens are also a smart choice. When shopping for fats in your diet grab some nuts, seeds, beans and legumes. The beans and legumes are high in fiber, and nuts are a good source of unsaturated fats. Healthy cooking oils are also a plus. Olive oil is the most recognized oil for its heart health benefits and superior amount of monounsaturated fat. No wonder Popeye had a thing for her. Additionally, coconut, flax, sesame, and safflower are also healthy oils to include in your meals. Think brown whole grains when shopping for good complex carbohydrates. Stay away from white bread, instant white rice, white potatoes, cereals, and baked goods with little to no fiber. Choose brown rice, sweet potatoes, quinoa, cous cous, buckwheat, and cereals made from high fiber grains to take home. Whole grain foods are less processed than white-flour based goods and are far more beneficial to your healthy and natural lifestyle. Below I've made a list of healthy foods, so you won't fail the next time you go grocery shopping. Don't let me down.

PROTEINS	VEGETABLES	CARBOHYDRATES	HEALTHY FATS
Chicken Breast	Broccoli	Sweet potato	Avocado
Turkey Breast	Asparagus	Yams	Sunflower seeds
Lean Ground Turkey	Lettuce	Squash	Pumpkin seeds
Swordfish	Carrots	Pumpkin	Cold-water fish
Orange Roughy	Cauliflower	Steamed brown and wild	Natural peanut butter
Haddock	Green beans	rice	Low-fat cheese
Salmon	Green peppers	Lentils	Olives and olive oil
Tuna	Mushrooms	Couscous	Safflower oil
Crab	Spinach	Kashi	Canola oil
Lobster	Tomato	Buckwheat	Coconut oil
Shrimp	Peas	Quinoa	Sunflower oil
Top Round Steak	Brussels sprouts	Whole-wheat pasta	Flax seed oil
Top Sirloin Steak	Artichoke	Oatmeal	Almonds
Lean Ground Beef	Cabbage	Barley	Pistachios
Buffalo	Celery	Beans (black, kidney)	Walnuts
Lean Ham	Zucchini	Corn	Cashews
Egg Whites or	Cucumber	Fat-free yogurt	Sesame seeds
Substitutes	Onion	Fat-free milk	(Hummus)
Trout		Whole-wheat bread	
Low-fat Cottage Cheese		High-fiber cereal	
Wild-Game Meat		Whole grains	
Turkey Bacon			

Vegetable Proteins
Tempeh
Seitan
Tofu
Texturized vegetable
protein
Soy foods
Veggie burgers

Fruits
Strawberries
Blueberries
Oranges
Apples
Bananas
Orange
Kiwis
Red and purple grapes
Papayas

EXERCISE

To this day I still don't understand how some people think they need absolutely no physical activity in their lives. How can you be physically fit, if you don't exercise? First of all, everyone needs to know the five components of fitness. Do you know them? They are **cardiovascular endurance, muscle strength, muscle endurance, flexibility** (which I need to work on), and **body composition.**

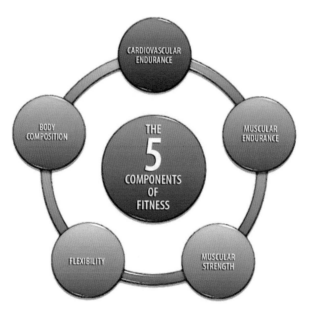

When you look at those five components, you realize that you HAVE to exercise to improve those components. However, so many people have reasons (or should I say excuses) for not exercising. Let's look at some of these common excuses and see why creating structure in your exercise plan is important.

In my opinion, the number one reason people don't exercise is because of time constraints. I don't know how many times I've heard, "I'd love to exercise, but I just don't have any time to." My response to that is "You don't find time to exercise, you make time!"

Take the time to study your schedule and find out where you can create time. Maybe you can focus on getting to bed earlier, so you can exercise in the morning. Many people turn their daily commute into exercise. If work or school is not too far, consider walking or biking to get there. If you drive, park far enough away so you can walk the remaining way. This is how you work exercise into your life, and why structure is such a key part of getting in shape. If you find yourself in front of the television watching reality shows, or playing video games, think about cutting back a little for exercise. If you have time for Facebook, you have time for exercise. Multitasking is another option you should consider. I actually walk the treadmill while watching my favorite shows. Focus on creating the time, and then treat that time like an appointment. You wouldn't cancel your medical appointment? What about your job interview? What about your hair appointment or tee time? Focus on finding an activity that you enjoy doing, make it part of your routine, and don't cancel on yourself.

Now of course everything you just read can only happen if you're motivated to actually do it. Over the years, I've come to realize that many people talk themselves out of being motivated. For example, you're reading this book, what motivated you to do that, think about it? Remember in the introduction I told you to stand in front of the mirror and think of every possible reason that you want to improve your fitness. Remember that? Well, use those reasons as motivation. You're never going to climb a mountain if you just stand at the bottom staring at it. Furthermore, you don't want to be sitting here a year from today, wishing you had started today.

The most critical part of any task is starting. Even though, it's a bitch to get motivated in the beginning. You'll come to realize that a lot of your motivation kicks in after you have started. I'll never forget walking into a gym while I was on vacation, and there was a sign when you entered that read "You've already done the hard part...getting here!" So with that being said, you have to create a routine you do before exercising. A very busy friend of mine created a great routine to get him started. Every night before he went to bed, he determined what time he could exercise the following day. He set an alarm clock near the front door of his home, and he set it to go off at that pre-determined time. Beside the alarm clock were his workout shoes, in one shoe was his bottled water, and in the other shoe was an energy bar. I would laugh at him, but he would always fire back at me with "Whatever bro, it works." So get creative and think of a pre-workout routine to get you moving.

Over the years another excuse that I've constantly heard when it came to exercising was, "I'm tired, and I just don't have the energy to exercise". To which my response was, "Guess what I'm tired of...excuses! The reason you're tired is because you don't exercise!" I understand when you're fatigued the last thing you want to do is exercise. However, as absurd as it may seem, expending energy by engaging in regular exercise will increase your energy levels over time. Research has even suggested that regular exercise can increase energy levels even among people suffering from chronic medical conditions associated with fatigue, like cancer and heart disease.

Now let's think about some of the things that could be draining your energy. Sleep is a big reason many people suffer from lack of energy. Think of your body as a battery, and sleep is like putting it on the charger once the battery becomes drained. Focus on trying to get the proper amount of sleep each night. Also take naps when the opportunity presents itself.

How many errands and chores are you performing during the day? Many of us work so hard during the week that the evenings and weekends become saturated with chores and errands. Cleaning the house, grocery shopping, studying, taking the kids to practice, all can become a physical burden as well as somewhat stressful. Prioritize these tasks, and rejuvenate your energy by exercising. Then you'll have energy to clean the house, kick the soccer ball with your kids, and sprint down the aisles at the grocery store.

Many people these days overwork themselves, are you one of them? In addition to the time spent in the office, many people allow their jobs to continue during non-working hours. Not to mention people being on call 24/7 via their smart phones. Learn how to compartmentalize work from the rest of your life, and you might find some new-found energy quickly.

Did you know that 55-65 percent of our bodies are composed of water? So many of us walk around slightly dehydrated, and that can really kill your energy. What's worse is that many people substitute coffee, soda, and tea for water. All of these beverages contain caffeine and many times cause dehydration without us realizing it. Remember to drink water throughout the day, and if you have any fluids that contain caffeine, increase your water intake.

Your diet is another reason your energy might be in the shitter. Eat for energy not for comfort, so make smart food choices. Also don't skip meals to quickly lose weight. Trust me this is a train wreck waiting to happen. This causes your body to go into starvation mode, which leads to your energy plummeting. Your body tries to conserve the little energy that it has left by storing all calories as fat and throwing your muscle on the energy fire. The result is, you have no energy to work out, and you burn up all of your hard-earned muscle on top of it. Remember what I said about eating your meals to spare muscle, because the amount of muscle you have does determine the overall speed of your resting metabolism. If you start losing muscle, your metabolism will slow down.

Here is another thing to consider when evaluating your time constraints. Our relationships with the people around us can really stress us out and consume time. Some people can just drain your energy and cause emotional stress. You have to recognize these people and put a little distance between you and them. Maybe it's that friend who is a time vampire, and they suck up all your time with a bunch of meaningless shit. How about that person who always wants to talk to you about their problems, you know the one that always takes an emotional dump right in your lap and you end up missing the gym. Find a way to reduce the effects of people like this because they will kill your energy, and many times bring you down.

Now that you've found the energy and motivation to exercise, the next thing we need to figure out is what type of exercise is best for you. This is important because so many people stop exercising because they don't enjoy it, or because they are not seeing results. Individuals who find exercise programs they enjoy have a higher success rate in accomplishing their goals. The successful exercise program is the one that is well suited for you. However, before you design a program, you need to know what elements to include in your program. A well-rounded program that includes aerobic, strength training and flexibility exercises is awesome, and will produce great results. Including these three elements in your exercise program will contribute to improving the five components of fitness. Also consider your current level of fitness, previous injuries or current limitations before engaging in any exercise.

First let's cover aerobic exercise most commonly known as cardio. Activities such as walking, biking, jogging, swimming, jumping rope, kickboxing, as well as others fall into this category. Cardio is a must for burning calories and paring down unwanted fat. During cardio your large muscles repeatedly contract and relax, which cause your heart rate and breathing to temporarily boost, allowing more oxygen to reach your muscles and eventually improving your cardiovascular endurance. In my opinion, cardio is a must in your exercise program. These types of activities lower the risk for many diseases, and have been associated with lengthening your lifespan.

One of the questions I always here is, "How much cardio should I be doing?" Obviously it varies with each individual, but I recommend starting with a weekly total of between two and three hours of moderate aerobic activity, or between one and two hours of vigorous aerobic activity. Examples of moderate activity are walking around 3.0 mph, bicycling between 10-12 mph, calisthenics, beginning yoga, and even mowing the lawn. Whereas, jogging, running, rigorous hiking, basketball, biking between 12-14 mph, and even shoveling snow fall under vigorous activity. Try and eventually work your way up to five hours of moderate activity, or three hours of vigorous activity for the week. This will net more results and added health benefits. If you're just getting started I would suggest walking, it's generally safe for all levels of fitness and age groups. In addition, walking is easy on the joints, and it doesn't raise your heart rate to dangerous levels. Modifying a walking program is as simple as adding time, hills, or distance to make it more difficult. Any of these modifications will improve your endurance. Just remember that a single aerobic exercise session should last at least 10 minutes, and make it something you enjoy.

Okay let's move on to strength or resistance training. This type of exercise involves equipment such as free weights, weight machines, and resistance bands. I always gravitated to this type of training because it built muscle mass. However, it also protects against bone loss, improves posture, and increases strength. It also improves your body's ratio of lean muscle mass to fat, which is another key reason you should include it as part of your exercise routine. Once again, I'm going to call back to what I said earlier, the amount of muscle you have determines the overall speed of your resting metabolism. Mechanically, strength training happens any time your muscles face a counter force that is greater than usual. As you build up to using heavier weights, and creating stronger counter forces for your muscles, the muscles naturally become stronger. When you start your strength training program you'll quickly realize how it also improves the functional strength needed to perform everyday activities such as walking up the stairs, climbing a hill, holding a baby while multi-tasking, bringing in multiple bags of groceries, or chasing after children.

Maybe you're familiar with strength training. Then again, maybe you have no clue what you're doing, or where to start. If you fall under the "I don't know WTF I'm doing category" then don't panic that's why you're reading this incredible book. Obviously not all of us have personal trainers, nonetheless there are some great classes and DVD's out there to help you out. If you belong to a gym see if your gym offers classes like "Les Mills Body Pump", "Bally's Power Flex", or any type of strength training group class. If you're training from home visit www.BeachBody.com and invest in one of the fitness program DVD's they have that focus on strength training. If you're planning on implementing strength training into your gym workout, think about the following.

First, allow 5-10 minutes for your muscles to warm up before a workout, as well as allowing the same amount of time for the muscles to cool down after the workout. Cardio is a great way to warm the muscles up. Many times I do a moderate cardio workout before I start my strength training, I either jump on the treadmill or stationary bike and knock out anywhere between 30-45 minutes of cardio. This way I've warmed my muscles up and completed my cardio for the day. A lot of people start working out with weights and become engrossed with how much weight they're using, and they lose sight of their form. Remember to first focus on doing the exercise correctly, and not on how much weight you're doing. Trust me, proper technique will lead to stronger and bigger muscles far faster than flawed technique. Align your body correctly and move smoothly through each exercise, if you're not sure how to do a certain movement ask someone for help. Shitty form can prompt injuries and slow gains. Start with little to no weight when learning a strength training routine, and keep your ego at home. Focus on slow controlled lifts with equally slow descents while isolating a muscle group.

Think tempo. Tempo helps you stay in control and not diminish strength gains through momentum. Try counting to three while you're pushing the weight away from your body, then try counting to three while you're lowering the weight back towards you.

Think breathe. Breathing correctly not only helps you take in oxygen and perform better, it also prevents your blood pressure from rising too much while performing strength exercises. The proper way to breathe is to exhale as you work against resistance, and inhale as you release. Does that sound easy? Well that's not always the case, so take time to focus on your breathing.

Think challenge. Finding the right weight to use will differ depending on what exercise you're performing. Select a weight that will exhaust the muscle you're working by the time you reach the last couple repetitions (reps), while still maintaining proper form. If you can't do the last few reps, choose a lighter weight. When you're at a point where it's easy to complete all the reps, challenge your muscles again by adding weight, or by adding another set of reps to your workout (up to four sets), or by adding another resistance training day to your week. Most importantly pace yourself, and keep perfect form.

Think practice. Working all the major muscles of your body (legs, back, chest, shoulders, arms, and core/abdominals) two to three times a week is ideal. You can choose to do one complete body (that's all the muscles) strength/resistance workout two or three times a week, or you may choose to break your strength/resistance workout into upper and lower-body components. In this case, be sure that you perform each of these components twice a week.

Think rest. Strength training causes tiny tears in muscle tissue, and the muscles grow stronger as the tears knit up. Always allow at least 48 hours between sessions for muscles to recover, the body repairs and strengthens itself in this time between workouts, and continuous training can actually harm your results. Always remember that rest days are critical to your performance for a variety of reasons. Some are physical and some are mental. Rest is physically necessary so that the muscles can repair, rebuild and strengthen. In contrast, building in rest days can help support a better balance between home, work and fitness goals, and prevent burnout. So, if you do a full-body strength workout on Monday, wait until at least Wednesday to repeat it. In this case, it might be easier to do aerobic exercise on the days between your strength training. If you're doing a partial-body strength session, you might want to work out your upper body on Monday and Thursdays, and your lower body on Tuesday and Fridays. This way the muscle groups you're training are getting the proper rest before you work them out again.

The last component that I mentioned should be included in your training program was flexibility exercises. Not only is it important to stretch after performing aerobic and strength training exercises, but it also important to have workouts dedicated to improving your flexibility. Flexibility exercises like stretching, yoga, and Pilates softly reverse the shortening and tightening of muscles that typically occur with disuse and age. Furthermore, these exercises reduce the risk of injury, improve posture, reduce lower back pain, increases blood flow and nutrients to soft tissue, and helps with better overall health and vitality. Always stretch when muscles are warm and pliable, with that being said, a great time is after you have done your cardio or strength training. Otherwise find another way to quickly warm up your muscles before stretching, such as a 5-10 minute walk, warm shower, etc. Another option is stretching between exercises, this also helps boost flexibility. Taking yoga and/or Pilates is also a great way to improve your flexibility while also offering a moderate aerobic workout. In addition, these activities combine stretching with relaxation which is great for relieving stress and improving balance (something we all lose as we grow older).

Now, that we've covered aerobic, strength, and flexibility training. Next you need to know what to consider when laying out the structure of your program. This is where you have to go back to that mirror and start asking questions. What are my exercise goals? Your program should include all the components we discussed earlier, but you may want to focus on a particular area based on your goals. For example, if you want to build muscle then focus on resistance/strength training followed by the aerobic and flexibility training. However, if you want to lose weight, then focus on aerobic activities followed by the others. Finally, if flexibility and balance are your main concerns, spend more time practicing tai chi or yoga.

What kind of shape am I in?

If you've been sitting on your ass for a while, it's impractical and dangerous to attempt to run miles on your first time out. Over-zealous people all too often wind up with extremely sore muscles, or injured. An injury is one of the quickest ways to sabotage any exercise program, and create an unwanted obstacle. Take it slow and look for activities that will create a more active lifestyle for you. If you've been a couch potato or a gamer, think about trying some exercise games like Dance Revolution, Wii Fit, Sports Champions, Kinect Adventures, or Wii Smooth Moves. This is a great way to get off the couch and ease your body into exercise without over doing it at first. Not to mention you'll have fun, it's low to moderate intensity, and if you have children they can play as well. Pace yourself and work up to greater levels of intensity as you get in better shape. By doing something more up your alley, it usually equates to fun as well as providing motivation. Remember, moderate exercise is safe for all, such as walking and light resistance training. Still, what if you're in pretty decent shape? Then consider doing activities that will present a challenge, or take what you're currently doing to another level. If you're really into cardio, and that's your main focus, then consider running, biking, or swimming in some races or events. If weight training is what grabs you, then consider doing a bodybuilding or figure competition. You'll find that training for an event can become very motivating, and it's a great way to jump-start your program. Just keep in mind, if you've suffered from a chronic disease or a previous injury, consult your physician about what you should and should not do before designing your program. This next question is important, because it's so instrumental in keeping you in check.

What do I like to do?

If you hate running, you're not going to keep up a running program no matter how good it is for you. On the other hand, if you love to bike, swim or dance you may find it easier to stick with an exercise program that's built around these activities. Remember to base your program on what you like, and not on what other people like or might be doing. Also consider your settings and surroundings. Do you have a membership to a gym? If not, then you might want to consider getting one if your focus will be strength/resistance training. What if you love swimming, but you don't have access to a pool. If that's the case, you might want to reconsider making swimming a big part of your program. Location...Location...Location is another thing to consider. Maybe you work in the city and you can hit the sidewalks for a brisk walk during lunch break. Conversely, if you're outside the city and your job isn't too far from a bike path or jogging trail, then that could be a good option. Study the vicinity you work and live in and decide what is doable.

Do I want to exercise alone or with others?

Many people love to exercise alone. They use this time to let their minds rest from conversation and to go into deep thought during their workouts. In contrast, many enjoy having others around them while working out. They find support, motivation, conversation, and camaraderie when working out in groups or with a partner. If you feel like you need a break from the outside world and want some time for self-meditation when you exercise, then you might want to work out solo. I have a lot of friends that avoid the gym, not because they hate the gym, but because they treasure that time alone. They invest in exercise equipment and workout DVD's so they can exercise from home, and they do their cardio either in the house, or they swim, run, jog or walk outside alone. However, if you feel like a partner would make exercising more eventful, and make you more accountable, then take group classes or find someone to workout with. Working out in groups allows you to be social, and be around a lot of like-minded individuals trying to get and stay in shape. If you like the gym, take group classes, consider Zumba, it's a huge success and dancing is a great way to get in shape. Finally, look into running clubs, or hiking groups.

How much money can I spend on exercising?

You really don't need money to exercise, just weigh cost against other circumstances, like the ability to exercise indoors or take part in a particular activity. Many exercise options are available at a range of prices. You can get great workouts for free by walking, running, or hiking. Try squats, lunges, push-ups, pull-ups, bear crawls, or burpees. All of those movements as well as plyometric exercises will not touch your wallet. Also, a set of inexpensive or used home barbells can produce the same results as a gym membership. With that being said, many people find motivation through the investment they make on equipment, memberships, and personal trainers. Not only can a personal trainer motivate you, but they can tailor workouts to your needs, and quickly educate you. Bottom line, if you're oblivious to exercise, elderly or pregnant, sometimes it's worth the investment to hire a professional to make sure that you're getting the most out of your exercise program, and not hurting yourself as well. Nevertheless, I do realize that sometimes money is tight. If that's the case consider teaming up with a friend or two to absorb the cost, or take a group class conducted by a trainer. Only you know what's in your bank account, and it may take some trial and error to figure out your financial comfort zone.

Can I push myself?

This is the question so many people ask themselves, and even the ones who have exercised for years. Another option to the personal trainer is the boot camp. Some people really need tough love, as well as someone badgering the shit out of them during exercise. Boot Camps were named after the physical preparation military troops go through at basic training. Not all boot camps consist of some psychopath in camouflage pants with a whistle around his neck screaming "Gimme 10 more push-ups, you candy ass!" Exercise boot camps have evolved into many forms and down many different avenues since they became popular 20 years ago. You can find boot camps geared towards, women, men, beginners, and yes, some for the crazed fitness fanatics. More importantly you can find the added benefit of peer pressure, and competition for those of you needing a push.

Before we move on to the next chapter, take this quick quiz to see how much you absorbed reading this Chapter on Structure.

Chapter 1 Quiz

1. **What three are considered macronutrients?**
   a) Fat, Protein, and Minerals
   b) Carbohydrates, Fat, and Vitamins
   c) Fat, Protein, and Carbohydrates
   d) Minerals, Water, and Vitamins

2. **What are examples of three good healthy carbohydrates?**
   a) Sweet Potato, Oatmeal, and Apple
   b) Steak, Potato, and Celery
   c) Salmon, Olive oil, and Beans
   d) None of the above

3. **What are the five components of fitness?**
   a) Diet, Exercise, Health, Age, and Progress
   b) Cardiovascular Endurance, Muscle Strength, Muscle Endurance, Flexibility, and Body Composition.
   c) Strength, Diet, Exercise, Endurance, and Flexibility
   d) None of the above

4. **A well rounded exercise program should include?**
   a) Diet, Running, and Sleeping
   b) Jogging, Yoga, and Vegetables
   c) Nutrition and Aerobics (Cardio)
   d) Aerobics (Cardio), Strength Training, and Flexibility Exercises

Answers to the quiz can be found in the back of the book

Remember, no one makes a plan to be overweight, unhealthy, lazy, and tired. That happens when you don't have a plan.

Onto Chapter 2

CHAPTER *two*

CONSISTENCY

One of my favorite stories is "The Tortoise and the Hare".

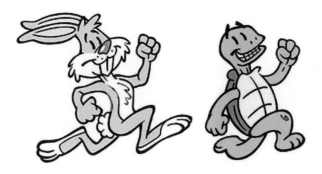

Remember, the cocky rabbit that never shut up about how fast he was, and bragged that no one could ever beat him in a race. Eventually he was challenged by the turtle, who probably was the slowest competitor he could face. Nevertheless, the turtle defeats the rabbit by staying focused, and not becoming distracted like his opponent. The moral of the story is "slow and steady wins the race." It's a reminder that no matter what the odds and how difficult the task, if you keep going you will get to your goal. The same principles apply when you're trying to get in shape and stay in shape. It's also the reason so many people fail with fad diets. Like the rabbit, fad diets boast what they're capable of doing. They boast excellent results, rapid weight loss, minimal effort, and in many cases no exercise required. However like the rabbit, fad diets don't promote consistency, and lack of consistency ended up being pretty shitty for the rabbit. In life we become what we want to be, by consistently being what we want to become each day.

Let's look at the word diet. What does it truly mean? The real definition of diet is "food and drink regularly provided or consumed." In layman's terms it means habitual nourishment. However, that definition has taken a backseat to the modern label that describes diet as "a regimen of eating and drinking sparingly to reduce one's weight" or "the kind and amount of food prescribed for a person or animal for a special reason". This is where I need everyone to reset that switch in your head, and define diet as "habitual nourishment". Remember you're eating because your body needs the fuel, and you're choosing what fuel to put into your body each and every day for the rest of your life. Get out of the mindset "I'm on a diet", because all of us are on a diet. However, only some of us realize that food can be the safest and most powerful form of medicine, or the slowest form of poison. Which way do you want to use food during the rest of your life? As a tool to heal the body and make it look and perform at a 100 percent capacity, or do you want to use food as a weapon to deteriorate your mind, physique, and health.

MOMENTUM

One of the first things we all need in our lives to maintain consistency is momentum. For example, a fist sized snowball can slowly start to roll at the top of a mountain, but once it picks up momentum it can eventually grow into an unstoppable juggernaut. With that being said, studies show it takes about 21 days to really turn a new behavior in to a persistent habit, and in my experience I would absolutely agree.

For example, I've always had a sweet tooth, and I remember there was a time where I was losing my mind eating desserts. Every day I was plowing down sweets, and it was a problem. I was feeling lousy, lethargic, and picking up a lot of unneeded weight, and fast. I knew I didn't want to give up sweets permanently, but I did realize that I had to step away from them to allow my body to break this crazy habit that I had formed. So for the next few weeks I had no refined sugar in my diet, only natural sugars from fruits. By the beginning of the fourth week I realized that I didn't have those outrageous cravings for desserts anymore, and I wasn't dragging and lethargic either. Eventually I brought desserts back into my diet, but only as a treat every once in a while.

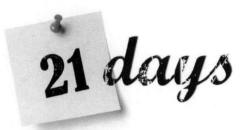

So 21 days people, keep that number in your head, because you're going to have to work diligently those first three weeks, so it can become easier beyond those three weeks. The hardest part is always getting things started. However, once you're moving, staying in motion and picking up speed becomes a lot easier. The key to building that initial momentum is starting with something you can easily manage, that's why the first chapter was so important. If you're just starting to exercise, start with shorter sessions and gradually increase the amount of times and the length of your sessions with each passing week. Some people make the mistake of biting off more than they can chew, and they burn themselves out before they start to pick up some momentum. The key is sticking to it, not trying to do it all in one day. The same applies to your diet, figure out how many calories you'll need to take in, and then how many meals you're going to consume per day. At first it might be difficult to eat perfect, maybe you'll need to have some white rice every once in a while instead of brown, or maybe you'll need a little more fruit to help with your sugar cravings. The important thing is you're establishing good eating and exercise habits, and you can enhance them as you get deeper into the weeks.

Another good thing to do is to find someone who can help hold you accountable. This can sometimes be difficult, because most of us can only take criticism from a select few. Many people can rub you the wrong way, when all they're really trying to do is keep you on track. If possible, find someone who knows how to motivate you the right way, someone who's opinion you respect, or someone who is also making similar changes in their life. This way, every time you find yourself thinking about skipping a workout or cheating on your diet, get in touch with this person and tell them why you are choosing to screw up. Ask for their honest opinion about whether your reason is legit, or it's just a lame excuse. You'll come to realize that this makes it a lot harder for you to believe your own bullshit.

Once you've reached three weeks and beyond, you'll realize that you'll still need momentum. The best way to do this is to set more goals. Whatever beginning goals you set for yourself, because you followed through with them, that will start the momentum. Furthermore, it will give you a sense of achievement. It's up to you, to take advantage of that positive energy, stay consistent and work your way towards the new and larger goals you've set for yourself. Keep in mind that your actions lead to results, which lead to you believing in yourself, which leads to you realizing how much potential you have. Individuals who have success also have momentum. The more they succeed, the more they want to succeed, and the more they find a way to succeed. Remember, one way to keep momentum going is to constantly have greater goals!

Another thing that kills your consistency is tricking yourself into thinking you are not motivated. I touched on this earlier in chapter one. The dreaded "I'm just not motivated (in a whiny voice)". Really, is that the real problem? No! It's not the real problem, unless of course you don't want to lose weight or become healthier. If you want these things, then there's your motivation, so stop crying about how you're not motivated.

Yeah I understand that, sometimes you might not want to exercise, or you might want to grab some fast food instead of preparing dinner. I get that, but it doesn't mean you're not motivated. It just means that you want two different conflicting things, and you have to make the right call. Convincing yourself that you're not motivated is just a way of denying that you really do have a choice. It's acting as though the situation is out of your control, and makes you feel powerless, because you lack something you need, the motivation factor. This is simply not true, and a bunch of horse dung! Furthermore, if you prepared your meals like you learned in the first chapter, you wouldn't need to make a meal when you got home, it would be waiting for you. Realistically, you would be putting more effort into trying to decide what would satisfy your taste buds. Driving to buy fast food takes time and effort, ordering a pizza requires waiting at least 30 minutes. You could have consumed a healthy meal, and satisfied your hunger in this time, always remember that.

Just be honest with yourself, and acknowledge that the choice is ultimately yours. When you're at that fork in the road, you have the power to decide which path to take. You can choose either option, without making gimpy excuses or whining out "I'm not motivated" to justify it. Then after you've made that decision, pay attention to how you feel about the choice you made, because the way you're feeling will play an important roll in the future when you revisit that same fork in the road.

Remember being consistent does not mean being perfect. You will have your bad days where you fall off track. Nevertheless, becoming consistent does give you the power to choose.

Another key ingredient in staying consistent is having a back-up plan, we'll cover this more thoroughly in a later chapter, but you do need to realize that life is unpredictable and complicated. Having a back-up plan in place is a very proactive tool.

If Plan "A" did not work. The alphabet has 25 more letters

You'll find that it serves as an alternative way to stay consistent when your regular routine gets derailed. I know you can't see the future, and believe it or not, neither can I (I'd be playing the lottery if I could). However, most of the daily obstacles that we're confronted with are ones we're all very familiar with. Deadlines and big projects related to work that expand your work hours. Feeling tired, lacking energy, or your significant other requiring your help or attention. The children or a family member is sick. Trust me, we all deal with these hurdles, the key is being ready to jump these hurdles as they approach. Put a little effort into recognizing the most common problems that disrupt your healthy routine, and have a back-up plan in play to handle these problems without giving up your diet and exercise routine.

Over the years, I've come to realize that consistently stepping on the scale can sometimes kill your ability to stay consistent with your diet and exercise plan. Seriously, it's like a double edge sword. If you step on the scale and you've lost weight great, but many times people use that as a hall pass to cheat on their diet. On the other hand if you step on the scale and you've gained a pound or two, then you're immediately frustrated and you feel as though you're failing. Bottom line, even though the scale is a way we can measure our progress, it can also be discouraging, and it also doesn't tell the overall story of what's happening with your body.

First of all, the scale can't determine your body composition. If you're losing fat and gaining muscle, then you're not going to lose weight as quickly on the scale, in fact you might pick up a little weight. It's not that muscle weighs more than fat. Realistically 5 pounds of muscle and 5 pounds of fat, is ummmmm…drum roll please… 5 pounds, that's a no brainer. However, muscle does weigh more than fat by volume. Fat is lumpy and fluffy and not as refined as muscle. Therefore it takes up more space, see the example below.

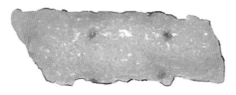
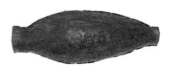

5 lbs. of fat   *5 lbs. of muscle*

Basically a pound is a pound, and it doesn't matter if it's a pound of feathers or a pound of weights. Muscle is much denser than fat, so often people misquote that muscle weighs more than fat pound for pound. The fact is a pound of muscle occupies less space than a pound of fat. So if you're losing fat and gaining muscle, it's not going to show on the scale. Nonetheless, it will reflect in the mirror and how your clothes fit. Also remember what we discussed in the first chapter. A pound of muscle burns more calories than a pound of fat, even when resting. So by increasing your lean muscle tissue mass, you're helping your body burn more calories. If you're weight training and eating a healthy diet that spares muscle, then you may feel like your routine is not helping you move down on the scale, in fact the number may even go up. However you will look thinner, and isn't that more important than what the scale says. This is due to an increase in lean body mass (muscle, bone, blood volume) and a decrease in body fat. Put your focus on how you feel, the mirror, and more importantly your goals.

The next dagger you can avoid is comparing yourself to others. It's one of the quickest ways to becoming inconsistent. Yes, it's great to use others as motivational tools. Still, too many people beat themselves up because they don't look like someone, or they are not progressing like someone. If I had a nickel for every time I heard "Why is so and so losing weight so fast and I'm not?" I would have money coming out of my a$$. Focus on yourself this is your journey, your life, your program, and your body. So don't lose your focus focusing on someone else.

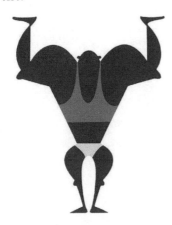 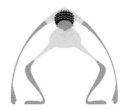

I'm sure you've caught yourself falling into the ever so captivating but emotionally troubling trap of comparing yourself to others. We usually do this trying to make accurate evaluations of ourselves. However, this comes at the cost of possibly positioning yourself in an area of self-doubt. Even though many people use comparison as a valuable source of motivation and growth, it also has disadvantages. The next time you're comparing yourself to someone else, stop and think…do you really have all the information. Do you know how long they've been working out? Do you know what their diet consists of? What kind of shape were they in before they started? Are they working towards a goal? How much time do they have in contrast to you? How old are they? Do they have the good fortune of great genetics? It's really not fair to yourself to make a comparison, especially when so many times you don't have all the specifics. Comparisons of you to others are both time-consuming and unproductive. Being hard on yourself actually depletes your motivation and decreases your chances of accomplishing your goal. If you really want to get in shape and become healthier, you need to dedicate your time and energy to your own plan. Your plan shouldn't be about being better than someone else, it should focus on bettering yourself!

In short, comparing yourself to others is a losing battle!

If that's how you're going to evaluate yourself, you will always be defeated. No matter how much you improve their will always be someone who is better in some form or another, so why waste your time and energy on that bullshit. Instead, learn from the talents and improvements of others, and transform that into creating the best version of yourself. So next time you find yourself using someone else as a reference point for your own improvement, stop and remind yourself how ineffective this strategy really is. Then graciously redirect your time, energy and concentration to your own goals and what you need to achieve them.

Your mindset is the biggest reason in remaining consistent. That's what separates someone who has struggled to stay in shape, compared to someone who has stayed in shape. It's all in the way you think. Your way of thinking determines your behavior, outlook, and mental attitude. If you think positive, you'll be positive, and positive things will happen.

What's your Mindset Today?

I won't do it

I can't do it

I want to do it

How do I do it?

I'll try and do it

I can do it

I will do it

Yes, I did it!

Can you Change it!

Let's say you're thinking "I don't want to exercise today." A slacker's mindset will think "I'm not going to work out today." Meanwhile, an individual with a positive mindset will think "I'll just do a warm up and get started. If I still don't want to exercise, I'll stop." Remember in the first chapter, I talked about half the battle was getting started. Well, the positive thinker realizes that, and puts themselves in a situation where the odds are in their favor to exercise.

Here's another scenario. "I missed all of last week exercising, and I ate a bunch of shit." The slacker's mindset will think "Well, I've already screwed it up, now why bother exercising." In contrast, the positive thinker will think more along these lines, "Damn, I screwed up last week. Time to get back on track, last week is in the past."

Okay how about this one. "I haven't lost any weight." Once again the slacker's mindset, or should I say quitter's mindset will be, "I quit, I'm just wasting my time." On the other hand, you the positive thinker will think, "If I stop now I'll never see all the results, nor will I hit my goals." Stay consistent and true to yourself. When you do something consistently, you take steps forward, without neutralizing your progress with backward steps. Commitment means staying loyal to what you said you were going to do long after the mood you said it in has left you!

INJURIES

The next thing I want to talk about is something that can impede even the most dedicated individuals, and that would be injuries. People who are just beginning to exercise are especially susceptible to exercise injuries, but they can also happen to experienced athletes. There are a lot of things you can do to avoid the injury bug.

Performing a quick warm-up prior to exercising is probably the single most important thing you can do to avoid injury. I know…I know, some of us are in a rush, and assume the body will warm up after we start exercising. Trust me, I understand it's tempting to skip your warm-up and jump right into your workout. However, is that time-saving decision wise, or is it asking for trouble? So many people take warming the body up for granted. They believe that they can quickly jump into their routines, and their bodies will be ready to go. This is not always the case, and that's usually when their workout is quickly brought to a halt via the injury bug. Below are a few examples of how warming up prepares and protects the body.

a. It will increase the flow of blood to your working muscles, which will prepare them for the additional workload you're about to put them through.

b. It will increase the delivery of oxygen and nutrients to your muscles, which prevents you from getting out of breath to early or too easily (many times, I started my cardio to fast and without warm-up, and it always lead to me under performing and growing tired quick).

c. It will gradually prepare your heart and circulatory system for an increase in activity, which helps you avoid a rapid increase in blood pressure once you start exercising.

d. It will make your coordination and reaction times better during your work out.

e. It will decrease the chance of you injuring your ligaments, tendons, and muscles. It's easier and much safer for warm muscles and joints to move through a greater range of motion.

f. It will help lubricate your joints for smoother less painful movement.

g. It will help to increase blood temperature, which can allow you to work out longer and at more intense levels.

h. It will start to activate hormonal changes in the body. Hormonal changes which are responsible for managing energy production.

i. It will help mentally prepare you for your workout ahead.

These are the many reasons you should warm-up before working out. Besides preventing injury, there are several other benefits you'll gain from a quick warm-up. A warm-up should be done before any type of exercise session. Usually 5-10 minutes is enough to get your body ready for exercise. Just remember to warm-up longer for intense work outs, and keep it around five minutes for the lighter workouts. Walking is always a great way to warm-up, or you can perform a lower intensity version of the activity you're about to do. Now back to injury prevention.

Don't overdo it! We talked about this earlier in the book. When you first start working out, or you find a new goal to target, you might be inclined to work a little harder, in hopes that you'll reach your goals faster. Sadly, you won't be consistent or making much progress if you're incapacitated because you went ape shit and pulled a muscle or tore a ligament. Remind yourself to slowly introduce your body to new levels of intensity. Remember my friend the turtle? Slow and steady may seem to take longer to produce results, but it's better than being put in neutral because you hurt yourself.

How do I know if I'm overdoing it? First of all, pay attention to your body. If you have any sharp, stabbing, alarming, or sudden pains during any kind of workout, you should call it quits for the day. If the pain persists have it checked out immediately. Furthermore, if you've worked a certain muscle a few days ago, but it's still sore and you're ready to work it again, you're probably over training and need a couple more days of rest. Remember there is nothing wrong with recovery day's. Muscles recover during downtime, not when you train, so you need to leave days for rest, recovery, and growth if you want to maximize the effects of exercise. Not taking advantage of these rest days, especially when your body is signaling you to do so, can result in injury. Other signs of overtraining can range from loss of strength, speed, endurance, or other aspects of performance during exercise. Also loss of appetite, insomnia, chronic soreness, chronic colds, and irritability are common signs of overtraining. If you have any of these symptoms and you've ruled out any existing medical conditions that might be responsible, then you probably need a break. However, consult your physician just for assurance. Keep in mind, overtraining leads to injuries, and injuries lead to inconsistency.

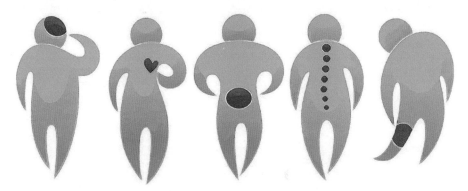

Use proper form when exercising. So many injuries occur from people using crappy form. If you don't know how to do an exercise correctly, ask for help and take your ego out of the equation. I don't know how many times I've looked across the gym and thought "WTF is that person doing! They're going to kill themselves!" Learn how to do each exercise correctly. The better your form, the better your results, that is a fact. The worse your form, the greater chance of an injury, and that is a fact. If you're unable to keep up good form, decrease the weight or the number of repetitions. Likewise, if you're running and your feet are pounding to the ground, or you're kicking yourself in the ass with each stride, you're using bad form. Also, taking strides that are to long while running can lead to injury. Always check your stride, if you're unsure about your stride, have an expert analyze it. Also, some exercises are just not meant for you. So many people force themselves to do a particular exercise even when they feel discomfort while performing it. Just because someone does squats in their routine, doesn't mean that you must have them in yours, especially if you feel displeasure when performing them. Consider other options such as lunges or leg presses. Realize that we are all built differently, and forcing yourself to do an exercise that doesn't feel good with your body, is not a positive. Seek out the exercises that keep you free of pain while performing and put those into your routine. If you've been running, and you find yourself feeling discomfort during and/or after running, then consider another form of cardio. The same applies to other types of cardio. Don't continue to do a particular type of cardio when your body is experiencing pain while performing it, it can cause agony, lead to injury, and more importantly discourage you. Once again, choose exercises you enjoy, and ones you'll find yourself continuing to do. Remember to train smart and use the proper form, even when you're warming up or replacing your weights. Proper form will protect you from aggravating old injuries, and lead to quicker gains. I would also like to add that you should always use proper equipment. Don't bail on the things you need to work out adequately and safely. Decent shoes, bicycle helmets, gloves, elbow and knee pads, and other type of protective gear is important. Even buying quality workout machines and weights is smart. I had a friend purchase a piece of crap workout machine. The machine failed, and left him with a broken nose after the cable snapped. I also had a friend that was biking, and took a fall without a helmet. That spill left him with a concussion, and about 4 weeks of down time from exercise. Taking equipment shortcuts is a risky way to save you a few bucks.

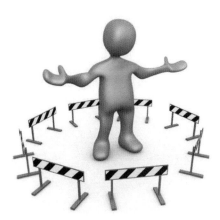

Use some common sense. Lack of using common sense has derailed so many people. If you know you can only bench press 150 pounds, then don't try and bench press 300 pounds to show how large your testicles are. Chances are they'll fall right off your body and roll down the gym floor while you're attempting this impossible feat. If it's your first yoga class, don't try attempting an advanced yoga pose that will have you leaving on a stretcher, use your brain. If you've never run over 2 miles in your entire life, then don't sign up for the marathon that's taking place next week. Always think logically and lean towards caution, you'll prevent many injuries and remain constant in your program.

Remember how important warming up is? Well cooling down is equally important. Just allow for a few minutes to bring down your intensity. The main purpose of cooling down is to bring your breathing, body temperature and heart rate back to normal slowly. During this time you are allowing the blood to properly redistribute itself to the heart. This redistribution of blood helps clear the muscles of lactic acid which can build up around the muscles during an aerobic workout. Stopping aerobic exercise suddenly and not cooling down can cause blood to pool up around your muscles in the legs. This can lead to inadequate blood flow and oxygen to the brain giving you a dizzy, light-headed, or nauseous type feeling. Therefore, always remember to cool down when performing cardio. After you've cooled down from cardio, or finished up a weight training routine, this is a perfect opportunity to stretch. Gently stretching out the muscle groups you just worked can go a long way in preventing soreness and strain. Plus it will contribute to improving your flexibility, which happens to be one of the most over looked components of fitness. Now that we've covered how to avoid injuries, let's discuss how we train through them. Obviously there are many levels of being injured. There are some injuries that completely sideline you, some that go away after a few days, and then there are some that linger. The ones that linger are a complete pain in the ass, sometimes they literally can be a pain in your ass. Nonetheless, these are the types of injuries we can often train around.

One question that I've heard come out of 90 percent of my clients mouths is "My [knee, shoulder, back, arm, calf, hamstring] has bothered me lately, but I want to keep working out. What can or should I do?"

Understand that being injured doesn't necessarily mean you can't exercise. In many instances exercise can benefit a person dealing with an injury. With some injuries, the injured area should be moved and not left stationary for a long period of time. Many people think that they should rest and not move the injured area at all, and sometimes that might be the case. Many times an injured area needs to stay mobile, and not moving it can actually make it worse. Keeping an injured area stagnant can sometimes lead to atrophy (the wasting away of body part). Always remember if you're unsure about your injury, or your injury is growing worse, consult a physician and get a professional opinion. This way you can make sure you're not doing any additional damage.

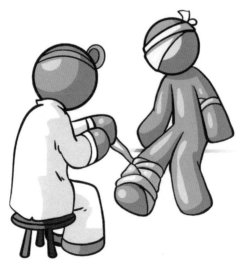

Once you've determined how severe your injury is, it's time to get creative with your exercise routine. If you have an injured knee, try to find resistant and cardio exercises that do not aggravate it. If you're not able to find any, focus on your upper body and flexibility until your knee has healed. The same thing applies for a shoulder or elbow injury. Find the exercises you can perform that do not aggravate the shoulder or elbows, and put more attention on the legs, flexibility, and cardio. Look, I've had several injuries over the years, and none of them kept me from exercising. Even if the injury required surgery, I did whatever I could to stay active. Then after the surgery I focused on rehab, and working the areas that were not affected by the injury. I always found that I came back stronger, refreshed, and determined. However, it was my mind-set that didn't allow these injuries to bring my workouts to a halt. I'll admit that my first emotion was frustration. I was down, depressed, and felt debilitated. Still, after deep thought I came to realize that sulking was not going to help my progress. Think about it, if you were driving across country, and you came to a detour, would you spin around and go home or stop driving? No, you would follow the detour until you got back on route, and then continue to your destination. A few years back I underwent hip replacement surgery. Leading up to the surgery I was in terrible pain, and it zapped my energy as well. So how the hell was I going to exercise, when just walking was agonizing and exhausting? Well, I hobbled my ass into the gym every day, and focused on my resistance training. I made sure my pace was very fast so my heart rate could stay raised as though I was doing cardio. I also managed to find a few exercises that didn't bother my hip, like leg extensions and leg curls. I continued this routine up until the day of my surgery, and after the surgery I took my crutches and went back to the gym. Staying focused and working out prior to my surgery had prevented my muscles from starting to atrophy, and it assisted me in healing and getting back to my normal routine much quicker. My family, friends and colleagues obviously know about my past surgeries, and there have been many. However, when first meeting people, they don't have a clue that I've had multiple surgeries within the last 10 years. When I share that information with them, they are usually amazed because there are no signs of it whatsoever.

Before we move on to the next chapter, take this quick quiz to see how much you absorbed reading this Chapter on Consistency.

Chapter 2 Quiz

1. **How long does it take to turn a new behavior into a persistent habit?**
   a) 3 days
   b) 12 weeks
   c) 12 days
   d) 21 days

2. **What's a good way to build momentum?**
   a) Challenging yourself with new goals
   b) Missing a workout occasionally
   c) Compare yourself to others
   d) None of the above

3. **What's a good way to avoid injuries?**
   a) Warming up prior to exercise
   b) Cooling down after exercise
   c) Using proper form
   d) Not overdoing it
   e) All of the above

4. **What should you do when it comes to exercising while injured?**
   a) Don't exercise until your injury is healed
   b) Continue to exercise just as you were prior to the injury
   c) Exercise around your injuries if possible
   d) Push through the pain of the injury
   e) None of the above

Answers to the quiz can be found in the back of the book

Remember, there are a lot of things that help us in this world to remain consistent. However, the single most important thing is your mind-set. Being headstrong will keep you focused on your agenda and away from bad habits. Speaking of habits, I think it's about that time.
Onto Chapter Three

CHAPTER three

HABITS

An acquired behavior pattern regularly followed until it has become almost involuntary. Yep, that sums it up, that in a nutshell defines habit. Our habits are programmed, and they happen without us even realizing it, and it's vital that we don't even realize it. That's the strength and beauty of our habits. We do them without even thinking about it. However, that's also the problem with bad habits. Those detrimental automated behaviors also run without us even being conscious of it. As a result, this can get us into trouble.

Our behaviors mold and define who we are, and habits are part of the groundwork of our behavioral patterns. If we can master what we build our behaviors on, then ultimately we can control who we are. Yes, some habits are destructive, but some can also be favorable. This chapter will cover the most common bad habits that prevent you from getting into shape. It will make you aware of their negative impacts, and offer you suggestions on how to conquer them. Furthermore, you'll learn how to change some of these bad habits into good habits. I know many of you have good habits, such as looking both ways before you cross the street. I've always loved that habit. It truly is a great way to prevent you from getting plowed over by a speeding vehicle, isn't it?

It's amazing how we involuntarily develop so many good habits to prevent us from being harmed, but when it comes to our bodies we struggle to create habits that will preserve our health. I believe that is because there are no immediate repercussions. Let me explain, if you step off that curb without looking both ways, there's a chance that a car will immediately hit your ass. However, if you smoke a cigarette, there is no immediate repercussion. Imagine if one out of every 100,000 cigarettes could cause immediate death. Do you think people would still gamble as much with those odds, especially if they turned on the news every day and heard, "In other news, over 51,000 people died today as the result of smoking a lethal cigarette." Fortunately there is no lethal cigarette, well let me re-word that, no cigarette that immediately kills you. Likewise, people continue to gamble with bad habits like cigarettes, even when realistically every 8 seconds someone in the world dies from tobacco use.

We will revisit cigarettes, but for now let's focus on the many other bad habits that prevent people from reaching their goals, and in many cases play an integral part in destroying their healthy lifestyle. To beat a bad habit, we first must become aware of what our existing bad habits are. Then once we have acknowledged our bad habits, we need to define what is causing or prompting that bad habit. For example, if you bite your nails or grind your teeth, what causes you to do it? Is it because you're nervous, maybe you're bored. Whatever, it might be, you need to find out what is prompting that habitual action. Finally, once we've acknowledged a bad habit and its trigger, then it's time to end it. When trying to eliminate a bad habit, a good solution is replacing that bad habit with a good one. As we cover the many bad habits that impede us in improving our fitness, think about if it's a habit you have, what causes it, and what can you replace it with.

LACK OF SLEEP

Sleep is a must for your health and wellbeing. Most people need between seven and eight hours of sleep at night to function ideally physically and mentally. Contrary to what many believe, the body cannot be trained to need less sleep than normal. With that being said, the amount of sleep needed for an individual can vary slightly. However, no one can continue to function at full capacity with lack of sleep. Even people who only sleep four to five hours each night will encounter some loss of performance. Not to mention, sleep deficiency can also impede weight loss. Recent studies have indicated that people who sleep less than 6 hours a day were almost 30 percent more likely to become obese than those who slept between 7 and 9 hours a day. Furthermore, there are two crucial hormones affected by lack of sleep, and they are "Ghrelin" and "Leptin" otherwise known as the hunger hormones. Ghrelin is the "go eat" hormone that tells you when to eat. When you are sleep-deprived, your body produces more ghrelin. So lack of sleep leads to your body producing more Ghrelin, in turn Ghrelin tells your body it needs more food. On the contrary, "Leptin" is the hormone that tells you to stop eating, and when you are sleep deprived, you have less Leptin. The result, lack of sleep produces more Ghrelin but less Leptin, which in turn equates to more weight gain. If you still don't get it, let me break it down in average person terms. Not getting enough sleep, screws up your metabolism, Comprende?

Sl👁️👁️p

How many times has this happened? You didn't get enough sleep last night, and now you're off to work. You skip breakfast because all you want is a cup of coffee to wake your ass up. While you're waiting for your coffee, you grab a quick breakfast sandwich or donut for some energy. Once you're at work, you're pre-occupied, and you keep going by guzzling down some more coffee. Works finally over, but now you're tired and just want to get home. Screw the gym, don't feel like cooking, I'll just grab some fast food, bang out some choirs and errands, then head home and hit the sack. However, when you finally find yourself back in your bed, you are too wound up to sleep. This type of day initially created from sleep deprivation can quickly turn into a dangerous cycle destined to wreck your health and fitness goals.

Initially lack of sleep will seem to bring no harm, and at first you'll be able to fight off the sleepiness. However, eventually you'll become sleep deprived and low on energy. This in turn will lead to poor food choice, lack of exercise, and ultimately unwanted pounds. If you're someone that is struggling to get enough sleep. Then try making changes that will help you get more sleep. One thing you might want to do is create the right environment to sleep in. Too many people use their bedrooms for eating, lounging, working, etc. Do all of that shit outside of the bedroom, and train your mind to realize the bedroom is for sleep, and for doing the nasty. Also don't eat right before bed. I know so many of you want to grab a bite to eat right before jumping in bed, but this can hurt your ability to fall sound asleep right away. Too much food cranks up your metabolism and can wire you out as you're trying to go down for the night. If you must have something close to bedtime, then make it small and low in fat. Create a routine where you're in bed at a certain time. Initially you might not fall asleep because your body will still be on its own clock. However, in time your body will become accustomed to your new routine and adjust accordingly. So try getting to bed consistently an hour earlier, and eventually your body will make the change with you. This is my favorite, take naps. I love naps, and they re-fuel me during the day. The body usually wants to take a nap between 1 and 5pm. If you're able to take a nap between these hours, or at any other time, take advantage of it. Even if you can squeeze in a quick power nap at the office, it will re-energize you and make you more productive. You honestly only need 20 minutes, and that will go a long way. If you nap for over 45 minutes, then you might feel a little groggy and out of it once you wake. Take it from me the expert, I often nap a little too long and I feel like I just had two drinks at the local bar when I awake. Moderation people…moderation. Another thing you should practice is controlling your worries before bedtime. Too many people go to bed with stressful things on their minds. Take time during the day to think about those situations, and don't leave them to burden you right before bedtime. Realize that sleep is an investment in the energy that you'll need to be effective tomorrow. A good night's sleep is something everybody loves, and why not take advantage of something you love that also benefits your health.

STRESSING OUT

Too much work has you tired, anxious, and annoyed. Mental pressure has you nervous, depressed, and angry. Whatever the case might be we've all experienced stress in one form or another, and sometimes that stress is a positive force. It can motivate you to do well at a job interview or maybe in a competition you've prepared for. Nevertheless, to many times we find ourselves dealing with the destructive negative side of stress.

Have you ever experienced sweaty palms leading up to a first date, or felt your heart pounding while riding a roller coaster? These are examples of how the mind or your perception can cause stress, which in turn affects the body. This natural occurrence has been with us since the days of our ancient ancestors, and it was a way to protect them from threats they encountered. When confronted with danger, the body instantly responds by releasing adrenaline, which elevates your heart rate, increases your blood pressure, and drives up your energy so that you're ready to deal with the situation. The caveman had these responses when hunting for food, or when faced with a predator. However, in today's world even though we don't deal with the same type of stressors our ancestors did, we still are confronted with challenges that make our bodies react the same way.

The way our body reacts to these situations is called the "fight or flight" response. When this happens our adrenal glands not only send out adrenaline, but they also send out cortisol. This raises blood pressure, blood sugar, as well as other things, and this is awesome if you're trying to fight off a tiger like a caveman. On the other hand, it's not so good if this is happening because you're worried about paying bills. Bottom line, having high levels of cortisol over a sustained time period will eventually tear your body down.

Stress is public enemy number one, and it's because of cortisol. Elevated cortisol levels will interfere with learning and memory, lower immune function, affect your bone density, increase weight gain, drive up your blood pressure, increase cholesterol, contribute to heart disease, and I could go on but I'm writing a book. The important thing to realize is that stress leads to higher cortisol levels, which in turn leads to deteriorating your health. It is a silent killer, and even if it doesn't kill you, it will destroy your body.

Before we move on, I'd like to go over some of the ways stress affects your fitness.

First of all, stress can leads to cravings. Many studies have linked the release of cortisol while stressed, to cravings for sugar and fat. Cortisol may also increase the amount of adipose (fat) tissue your body hangs to, while actually enlarging the size of fat cells. Most of us want that lean mid-section, a ripped six-pack showing off our abdominal muscles. However, you're more than likely to have a keg than a six-pack if you're stressed. Higher levels of cortisol also increase deep abdominal fat, so unless you're doing a belly flopping contest, cortisol is going to hurt you. Remember discussing how important sleep is? Well, stress can cause hyper arousal, a biological state in which people just don't feel sleepy, or are just too wired to fall asleep. Sometimes it might be a major stressful event that leads to temporary insomnia, or it could be chronic stress which could contribute to sleeping disorders.

Stress makes your muscles tense which is no good, and many times causes headaches. The hormones that we release during stress can cause vascular changes that leave you with a tension headache or migraine, either during the time of stress or in the period soon after. Tight muscles can lead to an attack of acute back pain as well as contributing to ongoing chronic pain in the back and other muscle groups. Recent studies found that people who are prone to anxiety and negative thinking are more likely to develop back pain, and studies also tied anger and mental distress to ongoing back pain.

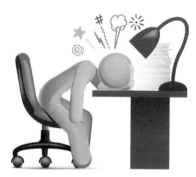

Remember back in the seventies an actor named Telly Savalas played a bald, dapper, New York City detective named Kojak, who loved to suck on lollipops. My mother thought Kojak was one of the sexiest men on television. She would look at me and say "I love Kojak's bald head!" That's great mom, but not all of us like bald heads, and even more of us don't want to be bald. Well guess what my friend? Stress can lead to your hair falling out. Isn't that awesome, you too can suck on a lollipop and solve mysteries like Kojak, all you need to do is raise your cortisol levels.

Stress is known to raise blood sugar, and if you already have type 2 diabetes you may find that your blood sugar is higher when you are under stress. Not to mention that, many studies have shown that emotional stress, anxiety, sleeping problems, anger, and hostility are all associated with an increased risk for developing type 2 diabetes.

Digestion plays an important part in staying healthy, and in helping your body use the nutrients it gets through nourishment. However, stress can cause heartburn, stomach cramping, and diarrhea. Furthermore, it can fuel irritable bowel syndrome, or IBS, which is characterized by pain and bouts of constipation and diarrhea.

Who the hell likes being sick? People who have ongoing psychological stress in their lives were less likely to fight off common cold viruses. Many scientists believe stressed people's immune cells are often less sensitive to a hormone that turns off inflammation, which could offer a clue to why stress might be correlated with more serious diseases as well.

Here's one I'm sure many of you know, or might have experienced at some time or another. Stressed out people have less sex. Not only do they have less sex, but they also enjoy it less when they do have it. Likewise, sex can help relieve stress. My advice, have a lot of good sex before you get too stressed out to have any.

Now that you understand how stress can adversely affect the body. Next, you need to identify what triggers your stress. Because I'm such a nice guy, I've compiled a list below of some of the more common triggers of stress.

a) Money or Financial Issues

b) Your Relationship

c) A Shitty Job

d) Taking on Too Much

e) Over-worked

f) Striving for Perfection

g) Continual Caregiver

h) Lack of Something You're Passionate About

i) Lack of Quality Time for Yourself

j) Pressure from Holidays

k) Unorganized

Once you've determined what triggers your stress, next you have to find a way to deal with it.

Worrying will not solve money issues, but it will make it more stressful. Take all that time you're losing worrying, and turn it into a part-time job. Use the stress as motivation to still change the areas you can, even if that means taking your ass to the gym to focus on your health. Relationships can spawn fights, arguments, and emotions that lead to stress and days upon days of being anxious and concerned. Talk it out with your partner, but more importantly be honest with yourself. Also not overreacting, and responding with compassion can solve many things before they escalate and become far more of a problem then they initially were. Ultimately, you know what you truly need out of your relationship. If your stressful days really outweigh your happy days, then you might need to do some soul-searching and ask yourself why you're still in this relationship. In any case, do the soul-searching while you're doing your cardio.

I love what I do, and because of that it doesn't seem like a job. However, I've had my clients that have stressed me out beyond imagination. Nothing is more frustrating and stressful than trying to help someone who is highly negative, combative, and doesn't want to help themselves. Eventually, I realized that dealing with their antics was not worth me being stressed the f*ck out. So I wished them well and severed my business relationship with them. Yeah I took a hit in the wallet, but in the end, the lack of stress and negative energy was definitely worth it. Many of us don't have the convenience of being able to control our work life. However, you can control your attitude, changing your perception of your job will reduce your stress and make your job more tolerable.

Some of us just don't know how to say "No!" I understand because I've been guilty of it way too many times. Sometimes you just feel obligated to say "Yes!" Sometimes you feel like you'll let someone down if you say "No!" Then, there are just some us that honestly think we can do it all, and cannot pass up the chance to try. In spite of that, nearly every displaced "Yes" we say, is really a "No" to ourselves. Not to mention this continued behavior can lead to you taking on too much and becoming completely overwhelmed and stressed out. You have to learn how to say "No" as hard is it may seem, you have to practice this. First, don't respond to things right on the spot, give yourself time. This will prevent you from responding under pressure, or reacting emotionally from the request. Giving yourself time to really think about the request will allow you to make the right call. Also try a yes-no-yes approach. First share with the person what you've already said "yes" to something else that is conflicting with their request, so "No" you cannot do it. Then follow that up with something positive you could do to aid their request. Here's an example, "I'm visiting my roommate from college this weekend, so I won't be able to help you paint your kitchen. However, I'd love to help you pick out colors if you haven't already found one." Just remember that by balancing your impulses to be a "pleaser" and "doer" with a responsibility to your character, you'll be stronger for it. Even better, you'll be less stressed, and more focused on the things that matter most to you.

In today's world the borders between work and leisure have almost completely dissolved. With new technology such as smart phones, laptops, iPads, and others, it's hard to compartmentalize labor and relaxation. If you're vacationing on a beach, and you're responding to emails from your boss, are you really on vacation? If Saturday night you're typing on your laptop finishing a work assignment while the family watches a movie, are you really having family time? Better yet, is it really the weekend? I understand that sometimes it's necessary to be enslaved by your job. However, that doesn't mean you can't conjure up new ways to balance work with the rest of your life, and recreate these boundaries that have slowly started to disappear.

Striving for perfection is not only impossible, but it's a major stressor. No one is perfect why in the hell do you think pencils have erasers. If you're never satisfied no matter how hard you try, or you're constantly dissatisfied with the people you live or work with, you might be adding unnecessary stress to your life. Wanting to excel and improve oneself if fine. Nonetheless, it becomes stressful when you're too hard on yourself or won't accept anything short of perfection. Many people worry too much about what others think of them, and this in turn can lead to self-hate, distress, restlessness, and isolation. On the other hand, you have a lot of people who are fine with themselves but are often frustrated and disappointed with others that let them down. If you're always badgering your children, partner, or co-workers because you're not happy with their actions or progress, then you need to take a deep breath and realize that everyone cannot always meet your expectations (and many times don't give a shit about meeting them). This behavior will only lead to tension, stress, and conflicts with the people you care about the most in this world. Trying to live without flaws can lead to agonizing times because it is often motivated by both a desire to do well and a fear of the consequences of not doing well. Perfectionism can sometimes be favorable when wanting to have higher standards or when wanting to work harder. However, it can also be unfavorable when it causes stress, emotional weathering, obstruction, and depression. Remember this on the road to getting in shape. You don't have to be perfect you just need to focus on yourself, stay consistent, and create new goals to aim for.

STRIVE FOR
PROGRESS
NOT
PERFECTION

Many of us have experienced or are experiencing taking care of a sick family member, an elderly parent, or possibly a child or person with special needs. Providing this type of care can place a considerable amount of pressure on a person, and caregivers are often surprised by the chunk of stress they feel. During these times you can feel financial pressure, isolation, fear, guilt, and complete burnout. When you're in this place it's hard to take care of your own needs because you're providing so much care for another. However, if you feel guilty for taking time out for yourself, think about it again in this perspective…How will you have anything left to give, if you're drained from not caring for yourself! Just remember to ask for help every once in a while, or accept it when it's offered to you. Stay connected with friends and family. Also find time alone so you can take care of yourself, exercise, and take part in things that you truly enjoy.

Since I just mentioned, "participating in something you truly enjoy." Let's go into that a little deeper. Our lives are jam-packed with responsibilities, and we often forget to engage in the activities that we're truly passionate about. It's important for us to feel more alive through the intensity we experience with passion. Those strong emotions that inspire us, make us cry, amaze us, and delight us are unwinding. Too many of us go through life feeling like something is missing. Take the time to partake in the things you're passionate about, and if you don't have any, find your passion. Maybe it might be fitness, or something you've never had the courage to try. In any case, finding your true passion can reduce your stress, as well as enhancing many aspects of your life.

Just how organized are you? Take some time and think about it, because mess leads to stress. Is your work desk a cluster f*ck? How about those dishes, are they piling up? Do you have a bunch of unopened mail lying around? Does the inside of your car look like a bomb exploded in it? What about your house, does it look like you could be on an episode of Hoarders? Being disorganized can lead to anxiety and stress in several ways. First of all, it floods your mind with several different tasks wrestling for your attention. Having all these different tasks on your mind can engulf your short-term memory. In addition, a crowded brain can lead to further disorganization by preventing you from completing tasks, putting you behind time, and keeping you preoccupied. All of this leads to your stress levels multiplying because of the unfinished business on your mind.

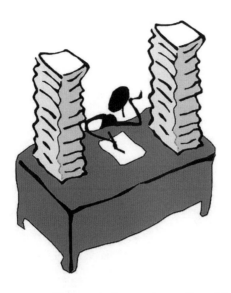

Being messy can also cause conflicts with the people you live with, and that leads to stress also. Many couples and roommates become involved in arguments stemming from someone not cleaning up after themselves. Finally, disorganization will drain the crap out of your energy. It's mentally exhausting thinking about the various things you have to do, and it's physically exhausting trying to play catch up. Don't put yourself in a place where you're wasting your time and energy wondering how you can possibly carry out all the things you let pile up. This will only lead to procrastination and more stress.

Take time to evaluate what triggers your stress, and remember that no amount of worry can solve a problem. I'm hoping this helped you become aware of a stressor that you might have overlooked. Moreover, I hope it delivered good suggestions on how to ease the various types of stress you might be dealing with in your life.

EMOTIONAL EATING

Feeding our feelings is a major no-no! Emotional eating is the practice of consuming large quantities of food. This food is usually comfort or junk foods, and it's eaten in response to feelings instead of hunger. Most experts estimate that 75% of overeating is caused by emotions. Many of us use food as a crutch to bring us comfort, at least momentarily that is. We often turn to food to soothe our emotional problems, and this is bad for a couple of reasons. One, it leads to unwanted weight gain, and in some cases health issues. Two, it's a habit that prevents us from learning the necessary skills to effectively overcome our emotional distress. It's a vicious cycle that starts out by a triggering event or situation. This trigger or situation causes you to experience uncomfortable emotions and thoughts such as negative feelings, stress, or lack of control. Then we wish to feel better and want to escape, we want comfort or maybe control. So what do we do? We eat to feel better, because these comfort and junk foods give us a sense of escape temporarily. However, after we've eaten feelings of guilt, disappointment, and failure start to kick in. We start to feel that loss of control again, and that we made a mistake. Once again we feel that desire to feel better, to escape, and we want that comfort and control. So what do we do? We eat more shit, and temporarily disregard our healthy eating efforts. This often leads to us completely giving up on our healthy eating plan. Then, we tell ourselves bullshit like "I don't care, and I deserve to be happy." Which we all know is a big barrel of donkey crap.

Emotional eating can quickly lead to being caught up in a whirlwind of hopelessness. By recognizing what triggers our emotional eating, we can substitute more suitable methods to manage our emotional problems and take food, weight gain and health concerns out of the equation. There are a lot of emotional triggers that cause this type of eating, stress, anger, boredom, anxiety, loneliness, poor self-esteem, and relationship problems are just some of the more common ones.

However, realize that there are other situations besides emotions that trigger this type of splurging with food. Sometimes it's a social setting that can trigger you to eat. Many times we find ourselves encouraged to eat by others when we're out at a social event, or we feel obligated to eat when others are indulging. Likewise, some of us eat to fit in, while some do because they feel inadequate around others. The next time you're out with friends take the lead and order something healthy, it might surprise you who will follow suit. Make your decision with confidence, that air shines through and many times causes others to take notice and do the same.

Then sometimes we eat because the opportunity is right in front of us. All of a sudden we're in this specific situation, such as walking pass a bakery with cupcakes in the window, or seeing an advertisement for a tempting food. Situational eating may also be associated with certain activities such as watching a movie or sporting event, or hitting happy hour after work. Many times these specific circumstances trigger us to reach for food.

Everything starts in the mind. Realizing this power of the mind is a very important prerequisite to being able to actually create the success and prosperity you want. In contrast, the power of our mind can work against us. Many people find themselves turning to food as a result of negative self-respect. We create these negative images of ourselves, and then use food to combat them. In some cases, we use the power of our minds to justify bingeing and eating poorly. Furthermore, we self-criticize because of our lack of control, and our defective image of ourselves. This only causes more emotional eating.

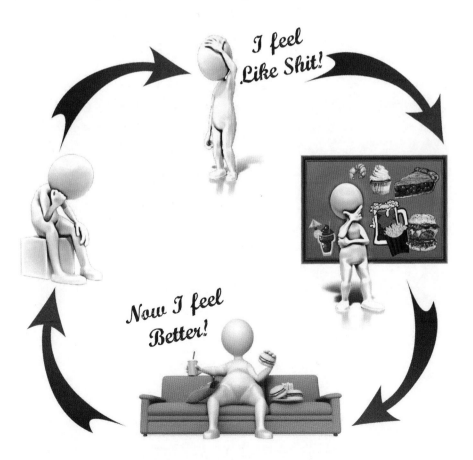

Finally, we have physical occurrences that prompt us to emotionally eat. Maybe we're suffering from a headache, and we feel as though food will cure it. Some of us skip meals, and then we get to the point where we just don't care what we eat, as long as it can quickly satisfy our hunger cravings. We're hungry, we want food now, and we want to feel comfortable while we're eating. For that reason, we created the name comfort food.

So how do we stop emotional eating when there are some many things that prompt us to reach for food?

First, you need to recognize what triggers your emotional eating. Tune into those instances when you eat but aren't really hungry. Then think about if it was an emotion, social setting, thought, situation, or the way you physically felt that lead to you eating. Ask yourself what's going on in those moments when you turn to food. If there's an emotion that's causing you to eat, instead of trying to suppress it with food, allow yourself to feel sad, angry, lonely, or happy. Too many people are afraid to just let the emotion they're experiencing run its course. If you've skipped a meal or you're really hungry, control yourself once you have a meal in front of you. Eat what your body needs, once you're satisfied stop there. Also avoid eating while watching TV, reading a book, playing games, or anything else that could be a distraction and lead you to continue eating without being aware. Finally stop and think about the positives in your life, and that so many in this world don't have the opportunity to conveniently binge on food. Furthermore, try to realize the irony in using a meal as a crutch, when in reality many of the disadvantaged need that meal to survive. Remember food is fuel not therapy.

NOT DRINKING ENOUGH WATER

Water makes up more than two-thirds of our body weight, and we could only go a few days without water before we would perish. The human brain is made up of over 75 percent water, while our lungs are composed of 90 percent water, our eyes over 90 percent, blood 82 percent, and even our bones contain 25 percent of water. Taking this into consideration, just a minor drop, such as 2 percent in our body's water supply can cause dehydration. Mild dehydration is also one of the most common causes of daytime fatigue, and research estimates that seventy-five percent of Americans have mild, chronic dehydration. This is a crazy statistic, especially for a developed country where water is readily available by tap or for sale in most stores in the country. The problem is so many people go through the day not realizing that they're slightly dehydrated, nor do they recognize the many symptoms. Remember this, when you feel thirsty, you're already dehydrated.

Did you know that drinking cold water can actually be a good tool for helping you lose weight? Yep, drinking cold water can temporarily boost your metabolism! A small part of this increase is due to the fact that your body works to heat the fluid to your core temperature. This spike in metabolism occurs about 10 minutes after consumption, and peaks somewhere between 30-40 minutes after drinking water. How much can that amount to over a year? If you increased your water intake by 1.5 liters a day, you would burn an extra 17,000 calories for that year. Those extra 17,000 calories would equate to about five pounds of weight loss.

Water is the most important source of energy in our bodies. When dehydration occurs, the enzymes in the body slow down, the result is a loss of energy and fatigue. Many times when you're dragging and you can't figure out what is causing it, it's the fact that you're slightly dehydrated. Guzzle down a couple glasses of cold water, and see if that rejuvenates you within 10-15 minutes. Many times when you're dehydrated and low on energy, you'll eat more trying to re-energize yourself. When in reality you could have just taken in some water and felt re-energized. When in reality you could have just taken in some water and felt re-energized.

Do you have issues with your cholesterol? Did you know that when you're dehydrated your body will produce more cholesterol to prevent water loss from the cells? Not drinking enough water can cause high cholesterol, something none of us need.

Remember I said blood is about 92% water? Well when you're dehydrated it's not quite 92% water, in fact your blood actually becomes thicker when you're dehydrated. This causes resistance in blood flow and leads to higher blood pressure. Not to mention, blood is responsible for carrying nutrients and oxygen throughout the body. Nutrients from the food we eat break down in the digestive system where they become water-soluble, which means they dissolve in water. Dehydration can lead to digestive orders as well. Lack of water taxes the digestive system and can lead to ulcers, gastritis, and acid reflux.

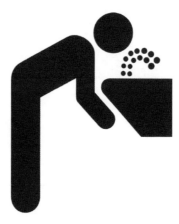

Water helps our bodies remove toxins in many ways. Water flushes toxins and waste from the body through urination and perspiration. Water helps reduce constipation and aids in bowel movements which ensures that wastes are quickly and regularly removed before they can become poisonous in the body. This waste buildup can occur in the body if dehydration becomes a regular occurrence, drinking enough water will also lessen the burden on the kidneys and liver by flushing out waste products. Additionally, a dehydrated body will cause accumulating toxins and acid waste, creating an environment where bacteria develop, resulting in the liver, bladder and kidneys being more prone to infections, inflammation, pain, and disease.

It's obvious that not drinking enough water really affects our organs, but what about our skin? That's another organ I bet you didn't even think about. You might be dropping hundreds on skin care throughout the year, however taking in a little more water throughout the day might produce better results. Dehydration causes the skin to wrinkle and age prematurely. Furthermore, it impairs elimination of toxins through the skin. With these toxins not being eliminated the skin becomes susceptible to all types of skin irregularities such as dermatitis, psoriasis, as well as discoloration.

Water serves as a lubricant throughout our bodies. The water in our saliva helps facilitate chewing and swallowing, ensuring that food will go down the esophagus easily. However, water also lubricates our joints and cartilages (soft tissue) and allows them to move more smoothly.

When dehydrated, the body is not equipped to send as much water to the joints. Less water means less lubrication, resulting in greater friction, which in turn can cause joint and back pain potentially leading to injuries, arthritis and even joint replacement. There are so many ways that water lubricates the body, have you ever used eye drops? Have you ever had dry eyes? Even our eyeballs need plenty of lubrication to work well and stay healthy.

On the average you should aim to drink around 64 ounces of water per day. If you're exercising (you better be), pregnant, breast-feeding, sick, or live in a warm climate, then you need to take in more than 64 ounces per day. Remember, the average adult loses about 80 ounces of water a day through sweating, breathing, urinating, and eliminating waste. That's equivalent to five pounds. You should try to take in more than you're losing, keep water with you as much as possible and you'll be amazed at the results.

SKIPPING MEALS

The habit of skipping meals is often seen as an attractive way to lose weight. Unfortunately, the negative repercussions of skipping meals are much more crucial than any potential benefits. For example, skipping meals can lead to your blood sugar dropping, insufficient nutrition, and your body metabolizing food slower.

When you skip a meal your blood sugar levels will decrease. This can cause several things to happen, none of them being positive. First of all, your body uses a series of metabolic processes to support normal blood sugar levels. When you start skipping meals, your body goes into a starvation mode. This is basically a survival mechanism that triggers your body to slow your metabolism. This in turn reduces the rate at which you burn calories in your body, which can keep you from losing weight. Additionally, your lower blood sugar levels can tell your brain that your body is hungry. This increases your appetite, and by the time you get to your next meal, you're prone to eat far more food than you need. Eating more at that next meal causes your blood sugar levels to increase quickly, and puts you on a blood sugar roller coaster. Not to mention, it will take longer to digest this larger meal because your metabolism is responding slower due to skipping earlier meals.

Sometimes blood sugar levels fall too low, and Hypoglycemia can occur. Hypoglycemia can happen when a person eats too little food, especially when they've been more physically active than usual. Often hypoglycemia happens suddenly and sometimes there is no explanation for why it occurs. When this happens, a person may have some of these symptoms:

a) Shaking

b) Fast heartbeat

c) Sweating

d) Dizziness

e) Feeling anxious

f) Hunger

g) Vision problems

h) Weakness or feeling very tired

i) Headache

j) Feeling irritable

Here are some tips to help you stop skipping meals. Make your meals part of your daily agenda, treat them like an appointment. Structure them into your day like we discussed in the first chapter. It is important to plan your meals and eating schedule ahead of time. Make it a priority to set aside a specific time to eat, and set an alarm 10 minutes before those times as a reminder. By following a plan we can start to gain control over our eating habits, and decrease our chances of skipping a meal. It is also important to listen to your body when it tells you if you are hungry or full. Keep a record of how long it takes your body to feel hungry between meals and make it a priority to eat when your body signals it is hungry. Ideally, a person should eat every three hours to keep your metabolism functioning properly.

One last thing before we move on. Did you also know that chronically skipping meals can set you up for the development of diabetes later in life? Try allocating an 8-15 hour time frame that you eat within each day, and try to have a meal around every three hours, but avoid skipping meals at all cost. It will lead to increased hunger, slower metabolism, poor nutrition, and in some cases diabetes. If you're going to experiment with intermittent fasting, make sure you educate yourself and get all the facts before starting.

ALCOHOL

People drink alcohol, some more than others, and some not at all. The truth is people have consumed alcohol since we stumbled upon fermented beverages back in the Stone Age, and in today's world you'll find people drinking alcohol for fun, stress relief, or because they simply enjoy the taste. On the other hand, some people drink because they're curious, feel peer pressure, or they simply want to lose their inhibitions. Drinking alcohol doesn't have to be a bad habit. If you're a moderate drinker, which experts define as one drink a day, studies have found possible health benefits. These benefits include, improved insulin sensitivity, cardiac function, and blood lipids (fatty substances in your blood, which when lowered, reduces your risk of heart disease). However, drinking excessively is a harmful habit that can lead to several health issues. Moreover, excessive drinking and getting into shape, is kind of like oil and water, they don't mix.

To start, your body metabolizes alcohol differently than the other foods and liquids you consume. Once you swallow alcohol, it travels down the esophagus into the stomach and small intestine. Your body quickly absorbs alcohol into the bloodstream, and eventually it makes its way to the liver. As the alcohol reaches your liver for processing, the liver places all of its concentration on the alcohol. When your body becomes focused on processing alcohol, it is not able to properly break down foods containing carbohydrates and fats. Here's the problem in layman's terms. Processing the body's fat and turning foods into sources of energy is a key job for the liver. If your liver is processing alcohol, it's preoccupied and the emphasis is not on food metabolism. Therefore, many of the carbohydrates and fats you've eaten are then stored as long-term body fat while your liver is busy processing the alcohol. End result, more body fat.

Remember earlier I talked about the effects of cortisol on the body. How cortisol caused belly fat, cravings, and other health issues. Well research has indicated that continuous consumption of alcohol over an extended period can raise cortisol levels in the body.

Alcohol is a diuretic, meaning that it causes water loss and dehydration. Along with this water loss you lose important minerals that are important for fat metabolism like magnesium, potassium, calcium, and zinc. If you're going to drink, try to drink a glass of water between every alcoholic drink or two.

Many people drink to lose their inhibitions, and even the people who don't drink for this reason, still lose their inhibitions. The loss of restrictions that come with drinking is usually damaging to your diet plan. Alcohol stimulates your appetite which is already no good. In addition, your willpower will be in the shitter when you're choosing what to eat, leading you to make poor choices. Likewise, your willpower will suffer as you eat beyond your normal portions. Your best option is to eat before you drink. It will prevent you from getting too hammered, and from binge eating.

Alcohol will also disrupt your sleep. Yes, alcohol might initially help you fall asleep, or you might pass out from being too wasted. However, the sleep you get is not the deep sleep your body needs to be well rested. This leads to you being tired the next day, which can cause the release of cortisol, as well as you craving crappy food. So the next time you're inclined to use alcohol to unwind after a hard exercise session, remember the unfavorable impact excessive drinking can have on various aspects of fitness.Controlling your relationship between alcohol and fitness can enable you to preserve your gains and continue to meet your goals, while also allowing you throw back a few drinks now and then.

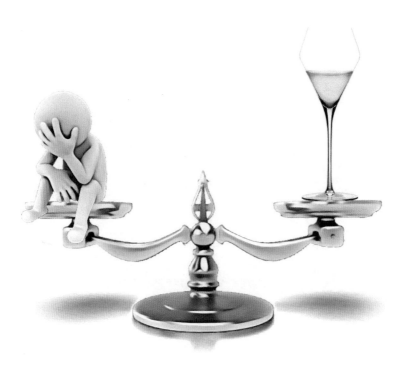

SUGAR

I have a crazy sweet tooth, if there is one thing that has always been my Achilles heel when it comes to staying in shape, it would be sugar. However, as much as I love sugar, I've realized over the years just how detrimental it is to your health. Not to mention, it's a habit that will surely prevent you from getting in shape.

I don't have to explain to you that eating too much sugar will make you gain weight, I'm sure you're very aware of that. However, are you aware of the other things excess sugar does to the body besides weight gain, and the storing of fat?

Did you know that consuming too much sugar can weaken your immune system?

Your white blood cells ability to fight off bacteria reduces when you overload your body with sugar. Sugar affects your white blood cells by challenging Vitamin C for space in those cells. As you probably know, our white blood cells need Vitamin C to destroy bacteria and viruses. The more sugar in your system, the less Vitamin C can get into your white blood cells. Meanwhile, the sugar is doing nothing to help your immune system fight off infections. End result, a weakened immune system leaving you vulnerable to viruses, catching a cold, away from the gym, and aching for comfort food.

Consuming too much sugar also contributes to diabetes, obesity, as well as circumstances linked to heart disease.

Over the past few years research has linked excess sugar to lower healthy cholesterol levels, and elevated triglyceride levels. During these studies people who ate large amounts of added sugar had lower HDL levels. HDL cholesterol is your "good" cholesterol because it helps remove LDL cholesterol (bad cholesterol) from the arteries. A healthy level of HDL cholesterol may also protect against heart attack and stroke, while low levels of HDL cholesterol have shown to increase the risk of heart disease. Meanwhile, these same subjects saw in increase in blood triglyceride levels. Triglycerides are another type of fat, and they're used to store excess energy from your diet. High levels of triglycerides in the blood are also associated with atherosclerosis. People with high triglycerides often have a high LDL cholesterol (bad cholesterol) level as well. Furthermore, many people with heart disease or diabetes also have high triglyceride levels. If you're eating twice as much sugar as nutritional guidelines suggest, then you're about doubling your chances of developing heart problems. Did I mention that the sugar is also destroying your teeth and aging your skin? So not only can sugar give you a bad heart, but it can also give you a smile like a jack-o'-lantern, and skin like leather.

So we know that sugar can lead to fat accumulation, but did you realize it also makes us to retain water.

Over indulging in sugar causes our bodies to produce the hormone insulin. Excess insulin production can "burn out" the insulin-producing cells over time, and this can lead to diabetes as many of you know. Likewise, having very high levels of insulin in your blood makes you retain sodium, a mineral that's found in salt. Whenever you retain sodium, you also retain water. Furthermore, excess insulin causes sugar crashes, which often produces headaches. So not only does sugar make you fat, but it also makes you retain more water than the Hoover Dam. Shit, I've got a headache just thinking about it.

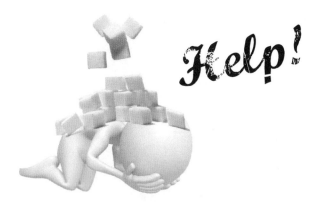

Did you know that sugar can cause mood swings and depression?

Once sugar is ingested (table sugar, donut, high carb meal, etc.), insulin is released, and it starts to direct the glucose in your bloodstream. Our brain cells need twice the energy as other cells in our body, and are extremely sensitive to changing blood sugar levels. The body in turn releases endorphins such as dopamine and serotonin to go with this sugar rush. When this happens we feel happier and a sense of calmness from the first intake of the sugar. However, the body immediately regulates the production of these hormones. Once the body has slowed down production of these endorphins, we experience a crash in mood, and in some cases mild depression. As a result, we reach for more sugar putting us in a vicious cycle to control our mood. This is why sugar is so highly addictive. There have even been studies with lab rats, that indicated that sugar was more addictive than cocaine. Yes, sugar is a delightful treat, but remember to have it in moderation so it's always a special occasion.

LOW-FAT FOODS

The low-fat craze started about 25 years ago, and today many people still believe that less is more when it comes to fats. I'll be the first person to say that being conscious of your daily intake of dietary fat is a positive thing. It's important in achieving weight loss, and preventing heart disease. However, like many things done in excess, it could be harmful if you take it too far. So you're walking through the grocery store and you see low-fat this, and non-fat that, and you throw it in your grocery cart because, "If it doesn't have fat then it has to be good for me"…wrong.

Think about this, if fat is removed from a food item, something takes its place to make it taste decent. In most cases the fat is replaced with high-fructose corn syrup, salt and artificial sweeteners, all of which are no good for you. Many of these low-fat foods advertised as healthy options actually contain more sugar than their normal (full fat) equivalents. Take the time to check the nutrition label, and you'll be surprised that in some cases, there is more than five times as much sugar in the so-called healthy low-fat option. Many of the popular cereals, yogurt, baked goods, snacks and ready meals labeled low-fat, actually contain levels of sugar considered too high by researchers today. Furthermore, many of these low-fat foods contain artificial preservatives that have been known to contain carcinogens, and these same additives can also cause severe allergic reactions and meddle with your health in many ways.

We also tend to over eat low-fat foods. It's like, once we see that label we lose our minds and assume that because it's low-fat it doesn't have as many calories…wrong! The Food and Brand Lab performed a study where they had subjects consume foods that were labeled low-fat, and others eat foods that were not labeled low-fat. The results of the study were very telling on how people view low-fat products. The subjects that ate low-fat foods consumed 50 percent more than the subjects who had foods that were not labeled low-fat. These people were encouraged to eat more when they saw the words low-fat, and in this study they averaged consuming an extra 84 calories.

Remember to pay attention to the calorie count on foods. Also check out the serving size, some of these little bags of low-fat snacks might contain 2 or 3 servings in one bag. Measure out single or small servings so you're not eating directly from the bag. Finally, if you think you'll be tempted to over eat low-fat snacks, defer and buy the normal version. Wouldn't you rather eat one serving of your favorite snack or dessert, as opposed to three servings of its so-so low-fat version? Realistically, it's better for your body, and better for your mind as it gives you no sense of deprivation. Assure yourself that with food, the quality is more important than the quantity, and be determined to indulge in sensible eating.

DIET SODA

I'm sure you've either seen this, or done it yourself. You pull up to the drive thru at McDonalds. "I'd like to order a Big Mac, fries, 6 piece nugget, apple pie, and a diet coke. That shit humors the hell out of me. You just ordered 5 billion calories of saturated fat and sugar, and for some bizarre reason you think the diet coke is going to save your ass. In reality it is going to save your ass, because it's only going to grow. The calories you're saving ordering a diet soda are irrelevant after plowing down fast food. It's seems like when we know we're not consuming any liquid calories, it becomes easier for us to justify that double cheeseburger and supersized fries. Realize that even though that chemical diet substitute has no calories, it's probably still is doing more harm than good.

Artificial sweeteners trigger insulin just like sugar. So if you're drinking a bunch of diet sodas during the day while you're sedentary, this can result in your body going into fat storage mode and eventual weight gain. Also because your body is producing insulin and not using it, you can become susceptible to acquiring type 2 diabetes or pre-diabetes.

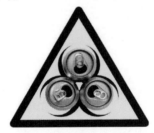

The University of Minnesota conducted a study that found drinking one diet soda a day was associated with a 36 percent increased risk of metabolic syndrome. Metabolic syndrome is a cluster of conditions which include increased blood pressure, a high blood sugar level, excess body fat around the waist and abnormal cholesterol levels. These conditions all occur together, increasing your risk of heart disease, stroke and diabetes.

Here's another thing to consider. When you're drinking a diet soda, yes you're getting no calories, but you're also getting absolutely no nutritional value. There is nothing in a diet soda that does your body good. That's why you're better off reaching for good ole' water. This way, at least you're drinking something that is essential for your health.

For all of you female readers, drinking cola (diet or normal) has also been associated with low bone-mineral density in women. Not to mention it leads to tooth decay in both men and women. As much as you may believe you're benefiting from drinking diet soda, the truth is quite the contrary, so give it up.

EATING TO QUICKLY

Most of us have very busy lives, and we feel as though we're constantly racing against the clock. Many of us scramble and rush around, trying to squeeze everything in throughout the day. As a result, when we stop to have a meal, we gulp it down and quickly get back to what we were doing. Likewise, some of us just gobble down the meal because we're hungry as hell. Guess what? If you're guilty of this, you need to stop and take time to eat your meals. Eating quickly is a bad habit that is stressful, and unhealthy. Taking a few extra minutes at each meal can have positive effects.

First of all, don't you want to enjoy your food? This might be one of the biggest reasons I eat my food slowly, especially when I'm eating something I'm not supposed to be eating…ha-ha! I love pizza, and every once in a while I treat myself to a couple of slices. If I inhale those slices like a maniac, it's a wrap… it's over…no more pizza for a while. I take my time enjoy every bite of each slice, and I get the same amount of great taste. Plus, I find that I get full faster when eating slowly. This happens because it takes about 20 minutes for our brains to realize that we're full. If you're eating your food too quickly, there's a strong chance that you'll take in more calories than you need before your brain realizes that you're full. There have been a growing number of studies over the last few years indicating that eating slower will cause you to consume fewer calories. These studies have even shown that you can lose up to 20 pounds during the course of a year by simply slowing down your eating process. Just remember that if you eat slowly, you'll have time to realize that you're full, and you'll cut yourself off from extra calories

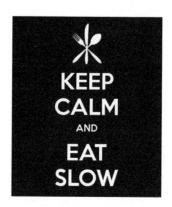

Eating fast also causes poor digestion which can lead to bloating, gas, and indigestion. Digestion starts in the mouth, and we need to chew our food thoroughly so that it breaks down

to a more usable size and state for the stomach. Chewing also ensures that there is enough saliva along with its enzymes mixed in the food to begin digesting it properly. When we eat fast we tend to swallow air with our food, which is a known cause of stomach gas and bloating.

As busy as our lives can get, we need to practice enjoying these little pauses we have during the day. If you're forced to slow down or pause during the day, instead of getting upset or anxious, try the opposite approach and enjoy these moments. The fast life leads to fast food, and ultimately to health issues. Slow down, savor your meals, and maybe add a nice quiet walk to the mix after you're done. You'll return to your busy life refreshed, energized, and more relaxed.

WATCHING TOO MUCH TV

I'm sure some of you are saying, "Why is this one on the bad habit list?" I'm willing to bet most of you thinking that, also have several shows recorded on your DVR.

When you're watching television you're being sedentary, and with the average person watching around 4 hours of television a day, this can lead to major health problems. Research published in the Journal of the American Heart Association showed that people who watched four or more hours of television per day had a 46 percent higher risk of death from all causes. This in contrast to people who watched less than two hours of television per day. In addition, they also had an 80 percent increased risk of cardiovascular disease. The body stops using its muscles and it can't appropriately process sugars and fats when you're watching television. This also applies to longer hours of sitting anywhere. It could be at your desk, or if you drive for long periods throughout the day.

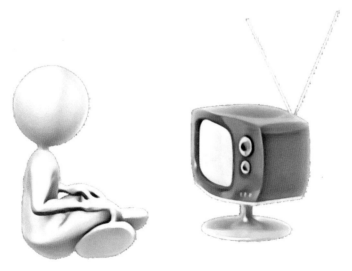

Prolonged, habitual inactivity can cause your metabolism to work at a slower rate. This can lead to your body collecting fat, as opposed to burning calories more effortlessly. Also think about this, if you're watching television you're more likely to snack on calorie loaded junk food. So now you've slowed down your metabolism, and you're snacking on processed foods that are high in calories with no nutritional value. Isn't that enough for you to realize that long periods of television watching is a habit that is unhealthy for you physically as well as mentally. If you must watch television, try doing so while you're walking your treadmill or while you're doing choirs like folding laundry.

SMOKING

This is a habit that I just can't overlook. If you're not a smoker, you can just skip over the next few pages (although you still might learn a lot). If you're a part-time or full-time smoker, don't skip over shit. Please read every sentence, absorb, and stop rolling the dice with your health.

My father was in great shape, or so it appeared from the outside. He had been an athlete earlier in his life, and had excelled in baseball and boxing. He managed to still have a lean physique, and played recreational golf until his death at the age of 55. Yes my father passed away at the age of 55, which in today's world is fairly young. He died of Heart Failure, also called congestive heart failure, and that is when the heart can't keep up with its workload. We all found it surprising because he looked young, and it never seemed like he was physically declining. I'll always remember the doctor coming in to tell us that he was gone, and then the questions the doctor proceeded to ask us. "Had he been sick...Was he a drug user...Did he have heart problems?" all to which we replied "No" The doctor continued on, and I started to realize that he was a little puzzled by my father's death as well. Finally, he asked the question "Did he smoke?" to which we replied, "Yes, about two packs a day" The doctor shrugged his eyebrows and said "That explains it". It was obvious he didn't have my father pegged as a smoker because of his appearance. However, once the doctor had verification that my father was a smoker, his bewilderment and questions ended. It was like this doctor had witnessed this over and over, and at that moment I truly realized just how toxic cigarettes were.

Nicotine is the hook. It is the addictive drug in tobacco smoke that causes cigarette users to continue to smoke. Habitual smokers need a sufficient amount of nicotine throughout the day to feel normal. In saying normal I mean, enough nicotine to satisfy cravings or control their mood. The more nicotine required of a person, the more smoke they are likely to inhale and this is regardless of what type of cigarette they smoke. However, nicotine is not the sole chemical smokers inhale. Along with nicotine, smokers inhale about 7,000 other chemicals in cigarette smoke.

I'm sure you've heard of the tar in cigarettes? This is the unified term for the different particles suspended in tobacco smoke. These particles contain chemicals, including several cancer-causing substances (carcinogens).

Then there's carbon monoxide. You know...carbon monoxide, that odorless gas that causes thousands of deaths around the world each year. Not to mention, it's the leading cause of poisoning deaths in the United States. Think about it, many smokers buy carbon monoxide detectors, and then defeat the purpose by inhaling the shit through cigarettes all day. I just find that bizarre.

Have you ever heard of hydrogen cyanide? Just the name should scare the living daylights out of you. Nevertheless, smokers ignore this poisonous chemical found in tobacco smoke. This and several other chemicals build up in the lungs, thus preventing the lungs from being able to clean themselves and remove foreign substances.

Then there's free radicals, these highly reactive chemicals can destroy the heart muscles and blood vessels. They act with cholesterol, in accumulating fatty material on artery walls. In short, free radicals lead to heart disease, stroke and blood vessel disease.

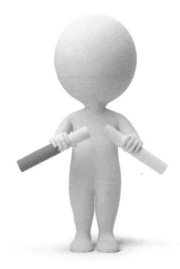

Finally, tobacco smoke contains metals (arsenic, lead, and cadmium), and radioactive compounds. All of these chemicals are known carcinogens.

Okay, I'm done preaching about what cigarettes contain, and how lethal they actually are. Some of you that are smokers will take my advice, some will give it thought, and unfortunately some will disregard it. Smokers disregard the warnings because tobacco is a gradual killer. It takes time to feel the effects from smoking, and because of this many smokers remain defiant. This especially applies to smokers that exercise and eat healthy. Smokers who eat healthy and exercise feel as though they're fit, and in most cases they've delayed some of the harmful effects typical cigarette user's experience. However, exercising and diet doesn't protect you from these side effects, it only delays the inevitable. Furthermore, smoking has been affecting their workouts, recovery, and overall fitness the entire time, whether they realize it or not.

Exercise places an increased demand on the cardiovascular system. Oxygen demanded by the muscles increases sharply. Metabolic processes speed up and more waste is created. More nutrients are used and body temperature rises. To perform as efficiently as possible the cardiovascular system must regulate these changes and meet the body's increasing demands. However, smoking has this effect on the cardiovascular system.

a) Raised blood pressure and heart rate

b) Narrowing of blood vessels in the skin, resulting in a drop in skin temperature

c) Less oxygen carried by the blood

d) Reduced blood flow to extremities, such as your fingers and toes

e) Can cause "Sticky Blood", which makes the blood more prone to clotting

f) Damage to the lining of the arteries, which causes the build-up of fatty deposits on the artery walls

g) The risk of stroke and heart attack is increased due to the blockages of the blood supply.

You need a healthy cardiovascular system to meet your body's energy demands during exercise. The above is the opposite. When oxygen isn't supplied to your muscles quickly enough, your body can't properly produce the energy it needs for muscle contractions. How about your respiratory system? You have to breathe to exercise, and those lungs need to work at full capacity. Nonetheless, smoking has the following effects on your lungs and respiratory system.

a) Reduced lung function and breathlessness due to swelling and narrowing of the lung airways and excess mucus in the lung passages.

b) Increased risk of lung infection and symptoms such as coughing and wheezing

c) Irritation of the trachea (windpipe) and larynx (voice box)

d) Prevent the lungs ability to clean waste from system. Leading to the build-up of poisonous substances, which results in lung irritation and damage

e) Cause permanent damage to the air sacs of the lungs.

Bottom line, smoking decreases your lung capacity, and you're not able to exercise as efficiently when your lung capacity is poor and your lungs are not functioning as well. Your body will perform exercise more effortlessly when it can get oxygen into your blood stream and bring it to your working muscles.

Smoking also affects your musculoskeletal system, immune system, and sexual organs. If you're trying to get in shape, and achieve better fitness put the cigarettes down, you'll get in shape faster and live longer.

Before we move on to the next chapter, take this quick quiz to see how much you absorbed reading this Chapter on Habits.

Chapter 3 Quiz

1. **Ghrelin and Leptin are better known as?**
   a) The sleep hormones
   b) Amino acids
   c) Fat burners
   d) None of the above

2. **What is associated with stress?**
   a) Lack of sleep
   b) Release of cortisol
   c) Loss of hair
   d) Belly fat
   e) All of the above

3. **Emotional Eating can be caused by?**
   a) Stress
   b) Being sad
   c) Being happy
   d) All of the above

4. **How much water does the average person lose per day through sweating, breathing, urinating, and eliminating waste?**
   a) 5 pounds of water
   b) 3 pounds of water
   c) 2 pounds of water
   d) 24 ounces of water

5. **Skipping meals can cause which of the following?**
   1) Hypoglycemia
   2) Increased muscle mass
   3) Better performance
   4) None of the above

6. **Drinking alcohol is excess can cause the following?**

    1) Raised cortisol levels

    2) Stimulated appetite

    3) A and B

    4) None of the above

7. **Consuming to much sugar can cause?**

    a) A weakened immune system

    b) Diabetes

    c) Anorexia

    d) A, B, and C

    e) A and B

8. **Low-Fat Foods**

    a) Often contain more sugar

    b) Are a better choice than whole foods

    c) Usually causes portion control

    d) None of the above

9. **Diet sodas contains**

    a) No nutritional value

    b) Protein

    c) Fat

    d) None of the above

10. **Eating to quickly can result in?**

    a) Bloating

    b) Gas

    c) Indigestion

    d) All of the above

11. **Watching too much T.V can cause?**

    a) Health problems

    b) Nasal problems

    c) Your metabolism to operate at a slower rate

    d) A and B

    e) B and C

    f) A and C

12. Cigarette smoke contains which of the harmful chemicals that can impair your health?

a) Nicotine

b) Tar

c) Arsenic, lead, and cadmium

d) Hydrogen cyanide

e) Carbon monoxide

f) All of the above

Answers to the quiz can be found in the back of the book

That covers it for bad habits. Now let's say good bye to them and this chapter!

Onto Chapter Four

CHAPTER *four*

OVERCOMING OBSTACLES

We all know that achieving our goals is not that easy, if that was the case we would accomplish them quickly and without adversity. Even if you have a complete understanding of what you're trying to do, and have envisioned how you will achieve it, there are…and will always be obstacles in your path. What gives us strength, motivation, joy and a feeling of accomplishment is clearing those obstacles on are way to succeeding.

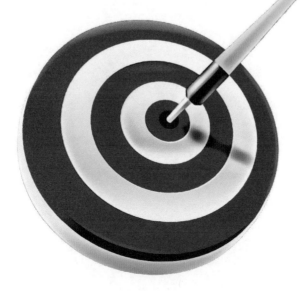

EXTERNAL OBSTACLES

One way to tackle obstacles is realizing the form in which they present themselves. There are some obstacles that are out of our control such as sickness, physical limitations, emergencies, business trips and dinners. These are external obstacles, and the key with external obstacles is to allow yourself to control what you can, and not worry about the things that you cannot.

We all get sick, so let's use this as an example. Catching a cold is an external obstacle, and for the most part we cannot control external obstacles.

We can try to prevent colds by eating healthy foods, exercising, practicing good hygiene, and taking supplements to boost the immune system. However, it's inevitable that sooner or later we will all come down with a cold. So how do you get pass this obstacle? First determine what type of cold or flu you have, and from there you'll be able to weigh out your options. As far as being able to exercise, if your symptoms are above the neck, including a sore throat, nasal congestion, sneezing, and tearing eyes, then it's alright to exercise. Nevertheless use your best judgment, and it's probably smart to scale back your intensity, because being sick can increase your risk for injury during a workout. With that being said, if your symptoms are below the neck, such as coughing, body aches, fever, and fatigue, then it's time to put it in neutral until these symptoms die down. So that means no working out, and no feeling guilty about it. Remember, when you are sick you need to take care of yourself and give your body time to heal.

Here is a question I'm always asked. "Kevin, should I continue to eat healthy while I'm sick?" To which I always answer, "Yes!"

When you eat a nutritional, well-balanced diet, many other components fall into place that keep your body functioning optimally. Foods that are full of nutrients help fight infections and may help to prevent illness. The key here is to make adjustments to your diet that will benefit you, and help you overcome your cold faster. Add some raw vegetables to your diet. They contain antioxidants which can reduce your chance of illness, as well as speeding up your recovery time from an illness.

Foods such as apricots, asparagus, beef liver, beets, broccoli, cantaloupe, carrots, corn, guava, kale, mangoes, mustard and collard greens, nectarines, peaches, pink grapefruit, pumpkin, squash, sweet potato, tangerines, tomatoes, and watermelon are high in beta-carotene. Vitamin C is also important and is found in kiwi, orange juice, papaya, red, green or yellow pepper, sweet potato, strawberries, and tomatoes. Finally, add foods that are rich in vitamin E such as almonds,

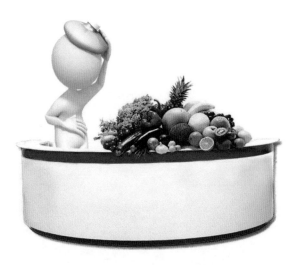

corn oil, cod-liver oil, hazelnuts, lobster, peanut butter, safflower oil, salmon steak, and sunflower seeds. Another thing to remember, protein is crucial to build and repair body tissue as well as fight viral and bacterial infections. Your immune system relies on protein, and insufficient protein in your diet may lead to symptoms of fatigue, weakness, and poor immunity. That's why it's important to have lean sources of protein such as skinless chicken, lean beef, turkey, beans, and soy in your diet.

When you catch a cold the easy thing to do is lay around feeling miserable while you shovel comfort food down your throat in hopes that it will make us feel better physically and emotionally. However, that's not the most effective route to take. Continue exercising if the circumstances are right, and don't let your cold be an excuse to eat a bunch of shit food. Make smart adjustments to your diet, ones that will help you beat your cold, and not ones that could trigger you into a bad eating spree.

Injuries and the physical limitations that come with them are no fun, and in many cases it derails individuals from the exercise program.

When an injury occurs it is important to reestablish some type of exercise routine, no matter how small or insignificant you might think it is. Bottom line, continuing to focus on your fitness is only going to help you overcome the injury and keep you on path to your fitness goals. If it's a serious injury, maybe initially it will be you performing your physical therapy exercises. On the other hand if it's less serious, it might be you modifying your routine to work around your injury. In any case, analyze your goals and injury, and decide what is feasible in both the short and long-term to keep you on your path. Design a routine that will allow you to regain as much function and fitness as possible. If you need some help creating your injury program, be sure to ask a fitness consultant, physical therapist, or other health-care provider to help you in this process. Too many of us forget that exercise provides several physical and psychological benefits. Refusing to become sedentary and finding an exercise routine that fits your needs and abilities can help you deal with your illness or injury.

Realize that coping with the stress of an injury requires both physical, as well as psychological resilience. Focusing on your physical rehab is important but it's equally important to address the psychological obstacles that can arise during these times.

People react to injuries with a range of emotions which may include anger, denial, frustration, sadness and even depression. Injuries and sudden physical limitations often seem unfair to anyone who has been physically progressive and otherwise healthy. Make no mistake, these feelings are real and are justifiable. However, it's important to move away from these unfavorable feelings and find more positive strategies to cope with this setback. Handling physical setbacks gracefully will help you to be more focused and resilient. Right off the bat, accept that you have an injury. Understand that you're the only one that can determine the outcome and your progression towards getting back to 100 percent. Be accountable for your recovery process, you will feel a greater sense of control. Also focus on the positives of recovery, rather than dwelling on the negatives of how the injury occurred or the setback you've suffered. Stay committed to your treatments, working hard, professional recommendations, and being consistent. Practice monitoring your self-talk! What are you're thinking and saying to yourself? Are your thoughts negative and self-defeating? If your thoughts and actions aren't positive, snap the hell out of it quick!

Furthermore, staying in contact with others as you recover from your injury is very important. Isolating yourself can lead to being depressed, and you're going to need someone to vent to. Plus others can offer advice or encouragement during the rehab process. Just knowing you don't have to face the injury alone can also be a tremendous comfort.

Finally set some goals, or readjust your current ones. Too many people use an injury as an excuse to give up on their goals. Just because you've suffered an injury, that doesn't mean you stop planning or setting goals. View your injury as a training challenge, as opposed to a frickin crisis. Set your new goals with the focus on recovery not performance. This will help keep you motivated, more confident, and moving forward. Continue to set realistic goals that are in line with your rehab and remember not to do too much too soon. It's easy to get a little overzealous when things are heading in the right direction, but this can lead to more setbacks instead of consistent progression.

One obstacle that we have no control of, and we're rarely prepared for is emergencies.

Emergencies can vary in size and importance, but one thing is for sure, most emergencies require urgent intervention to prevent a worsening of the situation. Therefore, emergencies become an external obstacle that can sometimes be hard to work through. In my experience, immediately addressing the emergency is usually the best method for preventing it from magnifying. My advice, drop everything and attack the emergency before it grows into something that could create even more down time.

Over the years so many of my clients have let business travel and dinners derail them.

It's a no brainer that cramming your normal exercise routines in between client meetings and business dinners can be challenging, especially when you're out of town and operating out of a hotel. However, unlike emergencies, you can still prepare for these business trips and functions. Here are some suggestions to keep you on track when mandatory work related events occur.

If you're on the road always pack your gym clothes and gear. A pair of gym shoes that can also be used as a running shoe, sports tops, shorts, and cold weather gear depending on where your location is. Having to run to the mall to grab workout attire is just one more obstacle that you can avoid. Also keep your bag packed with necessary toiletries to prevent downtime as well.

Do your exercising in the morning. When you exercise early in the morning, it "jump-starts" your metabolism and keeps it raised for hours! That means you're burning more calories throughout the day, because you exercised in the morning! Not to mention, you'll be energized, have a better mindset, and it will help regulate your appetite. More importantly, working out first thing in the morning ensures that exercise makes it into your schedule. Remember, you can't predict what will happen later in the day, a meeting could run over, a business dinner could pop up, or maybe a flight delay.

Find out if your current gym has a travel pass, and if they have a facility where you'll be located. Many gyms offer travel passes that permit you to workout at their affiliated gyms across the country. Even if your gym does not have branches in other regions, some health clubs will welcome members of other clubs that belong to the same professional organizations. If this isn't an option find out if your hotel has a gym, or knows of a gym close by that offers daily passes or memberships. Some hotels have deals with and partner with local gyms because they don't have

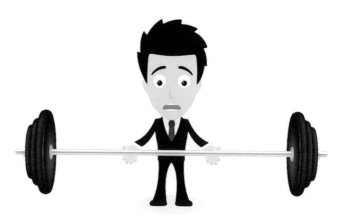

a gym, or their facility is the size of kitchen pantry. Finally, map out a walking/running route if you're out of options. Going for a walk/run and then combining calisthenics and/or plyometrics will definitely provide a great calorie burning workout.

Remember there's a flip side to this coin, and that's planning ahead so it's easier to adhere to your healthy diet.

When I travel I always try to choose a place that has a kitchen like the Residence Inn at Marriott. Upon arriving I use my first opportunity to do some healthy grocery shopping. This way I always have the option of cooking a healthy meal in my hotel room. Nevertheless, I realize that far too many times this is not an option, and you're forced to eat out. First of all, most restaurants have healthy options. So whether you're out at a restaurant for a business function, or you're grabbing something for takeout, make sure you review the healthy options. Too many times we let stress and foreign environments decide what we eat. Don't let the stress of travel derail you, especially when you have healthy options sitting right in front of you. Also pack healthy snacks such as protein bars, nuts, and even turkey jerky. These can serve as your go to foods in between meals. They'll help regulate your hunger and blood sugar. More importantly, they'll keep you away from getting stranded with unhealthy vending machine options.

Also reward yourself. It's nice and comforting to know that you have something to look forward to after a stressful day of work. Why not enjoy a nice healthy dinner to help you unwind from a busy day.

Decide ahead of time to stick to your healthy routine. Try working out early and packing healthy snacks, plus make healthier meal choices when the opportunity presents itself.

INTERNAL OBSTACLES

There are also obstacles like not being motivated, time, money, confidence, or just being tired. These are internal obstacles, and you actually have direct control over these obstacles.

Lack of motivation is probably the biggest and most common internal obstacle people deal with. Not only is it hard to get motivated, it's also hard to stay motivated.

One way to get motivated is to psych yourself up, instead of psyching your out. Put yourself in the shoes of your favorite athlete, or someone you admire for their fitness. Imagine their regimen, consistency and dedication, put yourself in that driven mindset and get going.

Find a picture of yourself at your heaviest, and take a good look at it. Think about how it makes you feel. Then find one of yourself at your thinnest, take a good look at it, how does it make you feel? Think about which one motivates you more. This way you can determine what motivates and drives you more, is it the negative or the positive picture? Once you've determined what motivates you more, find some additional pictures and strategically place them where it matters. Post them in the pantry, on the fridge, and by your alarm clock, as a reminder not to hit that "snooze" button! Open up a fit bank account, or buy a fit piggy bank. Then every time you make a positive fitness decision, drop a dollar in the bank. It could be declining dessert, or making it to the gym when you were telling yourself not to go. In any case, reward yourself by dropping a dollar in your bank when you overcome a fitness obstacle. Then once you've accumulated some cash, treat yourself to some new exercise gear.

Visuals are great for overcoming internal obstacles while providing that motivation you need to keep moving forward.

Write down your goals, and place them where they'll be a constant reminder of what you're trying to achieve. Creating accountability charts that consist of your weekly and monthly fitness goals is also another great idea.

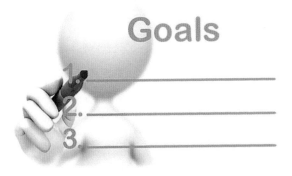

Do you have clothes or perhaps some jeans that you want to fit in? Well try slipping them on every time you have the urge to eat something shitty. If you need pliers to pull up the zipper, you'll probably think twice before chowing down on that cookie or ice cream. Then take those same jeans and stick them in the pantry if you have to. Trust me, doing this will serve as a valuable tool for preventing you from going down that emotional eating path. Furthermore, it will remind you that no food tastes as good, as thin and healthy feels.

Finally, strip down butt naked and stand in front of the mirror. How many times have you been trying on clothes in a dressing room, and not been satisfied by what you saw in that mirror? The mirror is far more honest and accurate then the scale. It will truly show you where you stand, and more times than none it will motivate your ass right out the door and to the gym. So while you're standing there looking in the mirror, remind yourself aloud why you're not going to binge eat, and why you are going to go exercise. Emphasize to yourself that you're on a journey, and you will not succumb to emotional eating. Alternatively, you'll create motivation and fitspiration to bring you one step closer to meeting your goals.

Chaotic schedules and full-time jobs are challenging. However, don't let time constraints become an obstacle getting in the way of your weight loss program. Try these suggestions to get past the roadblocks.

One of the most important aspects of an efficient schedule is planning ahead. Plan your workout week ahead of time, and treat your workouts like mandatory appointments. Sunday evening is the perfect time to lay out all of your exercise sessions for the upcoming week. Also include a couple extra weekend time slots for when life throws an unexpected external obstacle at you. You can also use this time to plan a week's worth of quick, travel-friendly meals. Bringing prepared meals during the day means you have more control over how many calories you'll consume. Furthermore, preparing your meals creates more time, time that you wouldn't have if you had to go out for meal. This extra time can equate to using your lunch break as time to exercise.

Another thing to consider is keeping some non-perishable healthy breakfast options at work. Sometimes, we rush out the door without breakfast, and that can lead to quick unhealthy fixes once your appetite builds up. Keep fresh fruit, quick oats, or cream of wheat at your place of work. This way you have a healthy option waiting for you at work, all you need is some hot water and you're in business. Surprisingly, many times overwhelmed people have congested schedules due to lack of organization, and not because they have a crazy workload. So remember to plan ahead to prevent unneeded time constraints.

So many of us are not morning people, and we have this ongoing affair with our snooze button. Even the ones who are morning people still struggle with exercising first thing in the morning. Nevertheless, exercising at the crack of dawn is a guarantee that you'll get it in. It protects you from being derailed by unexpected congestion and the excuses that are sure to follow. Initially it's challenging and many struggle with getting up and immediately heading off to exercise. However, your body quickly gets use to it, and you find that it's invigorating and a great jump-start to your day. Best of all, it's behind you so the kids, late meetings, evening events, and happy hour with colleagues can't get in the way.

The more convenient it is to exercise, the more likely it will happen.

Find a gym that is a rock throw away from where you work. This makes it convenient to quickly pop into the gym before work, during your lunch break, or after you get off. It also can put you in view of other exercisers which can offer motivation. Consider renting a locker at the gym, this way you'll have everything you need for a workout at the facility. This will eliminate the "I don't have my gym shit" excuse and help you stick to your game plan. Also think about asking one of your co-workers if they want to go to gym or exercise with you. Having a fitness companion to rely on can really help get you in a rhythm and keep you motivated. Exercising with a friend can provide new challenges, workouts, and keep your routine fresh and exciting!

Whether it's turning your commute into a workout or multi-tasking on the treadmill, being prepared and resourceful goes a long way in creating time for your fitness.

Improving your fitness can get expensive, hmmm? Gym memberships, healthy food, and workout gear can put a dent in your wallet? Really, let's look at that closely and go over your options.

Before I start remember this. The cost of poor health, low self-esteem, and an unfulfilled life is far greater than the cost of improving your fitness.

First of all you don't need a gym membership to get into shape. Walking, running, and jogging are some of the best forms of exercise out there, and it doesn't cost anything. They all provide fat burning cardio while toning the muscles, and strengthening the heart and lungs. Remember, there was a time when treadmills were not an option, and taking a walk, run or jog actually meant getting outside and enjoying some scenery.

Biking is another effective way to get a great workout. Put the spinning class/stationary bike on pause and move your cycling workout to the great outdoors. Cycling outdoors has its benefits, you'll find that time passes faster due to the refreshing distraction of scenery. The outdoor scenery also tends to draw your attention away from the challenging parts of the ride, which equates to a more effective and enjoyable workout. Cycling outdoors also works the glutes (butt muscles), hamstrings, quadriceps, shins and calves harder than indoor cycling. In-line skating also known as rollerblading also burns loads of calories. Moreover, it tones and tightens the leg and butt muscles.

Another great combination of strength-building and cardiovascular exercise is hiking. Hiking can burn almost as many calories as jogging. It's challenging and you get a good sweat going while enjoying the benefits of calming sights, sounds of nature, and a stress free environment (unless a bear is chasing you). Hiking works the butt, legs, abs, and it builds cardiovascular endurance. To really focus on those muscles and burn a ton of calories, choose a hiking territory with some hilly terrain.

NO GYM REQUIRED!

Another great alternative to the gym is doing calisthenics. I'm sure you're all familiar with calisthenics. Well there's a reason they're used to improve conditioning in sports and physical education. It's because they're highly effective, and have proven results. Calisthenics can benefit both muscular and cardiovascular fitness, in addition to improving psychomotor skills such as balance, agility and coordination. Calisthenics consists of workouts that use your own bodyweight as resistance. All you need is adequate space and these workouts can be carried out just about anywhere. The following are some great examples of calisthenics. I'm sure you're familiar with most of them, but if you're not, here ya go.

Sit-ups/Crunches

Start with your back on the floor, knees bent, bottoms of your feet against the floor. Lift shoulders off the floor by tightening abdominal muscles bringing your chest closer to your knees. Then slowly lower back to the floor with a smooth movement.

Leg Raise

Lie down flat on your back with your hands under your lower back. Slowly raise your legs a few inches off the floor. Lifting your legs slowly prevent you from gaining momentum from the upwards swing. Also, the slower you raise your legs, the more work your muscles must do resulting in a better work-out. Slowly lower your feet to the floor without your heels touching the floor, then repeat.

Jumping Jacks

Stand with feet together, knees slightly bent, and arms to sides. Jump while raising arms and separating legs to sides. Land on the balls of your feet with your arms extended overhead. Jump again while lowering arms and returning legs to midline.

Push-ups

Start face down on floor, palms against floor under shoulders, toes curled up against floor. Push up with arms keeping a straight line from head through toes. Lower to within a few inches off floor and repeat. You should keep your head tilted upward, and back straight. Do not rest on your shoulder blades, even when you feel fatigue.

Squats

Stand with feet shoulder width apart. Squat down so your thighs are parallel to the floor bringing your arms forward and parallel to the floor as well. Return to standing position. Repeat. Again, if you feel like this is not a challenge, there are other forms of squats. One method is lifting one leg off the floor in front of you, putting both arms in front of you for balance, and squatting. This is a one-legged squat or pistol. Squats are deemed by many health experts as unsafe, because they put too much stress on the knee joints. So if you have any knee issues, you might want to exclude this exercise in your routine.

Lunges

Lunges are a leg work out that enhances flexibility, balance, mobility, and muscle endurance. To carry out lunges, stand with your feet alongside one another and your hands by your sides. Take a big step forward, bend your legs and lower your rear knee to the ground. Push off your front leg to go back to the beginning position. Standing in the upright position, execute one more rep leading with the opposing leg. Keep on switching legs for the entire length of the set.

Pull-ups/Chin-ups

Pull-ups and chin-ups are two of the more demanding calisthenics exercises. They focus on your upper back and biceps muscles. To carry out these workouts, hang from a resilient overhead bar. Then from a completely extended posture, bend your arms and pull yourself up so that your chin is over the bar. Gradually lower yourself back down to the beginning posture and do it again. Pull-ups are conducted with a wider than shoulder-width grip while Chin-ups are carried out with an underhand grip. These workouts can be performed easier positioning your feet on a chair underneath you thus using your feet as assistance.

Plyometrics is another substitute to the gym. Plyometrics also known as jump training is an exercising technique that increases muscular power and explosiveness. It was originally developed for Olympic athletes, but now plyometric training has become a popular workout routine for people of all ages, including children and adolescents. Best part, you don't need a gym to do these fat burning exercises. The following are some examples of some popular plyometric exercises. Some require a medicine ball, but purchasing one shouldn't make you go broke.

Burpees

Incredibly similar to squat thrusts, burpees are performed without weights and require the individual to jump at the end of the exercise and not simply stand up. Start by standing upright with the feet together. Squat down into and extend the legs into a push-up position. Perform a push-up, bring the legs back toward the body, and jump straight up. Repeat this motion.

Squat Jumps

Using a similar motion to the squat exercise, squat jumps require one to bend their knees into a squatting motion before leaping directly vertical, fully extending their arms and legs (with toes pointed). Lower the arms and bend the knees as you descend back down and repeat the motion.

Tuck Jumps

Standing with both feet together, jump straight up bringing your knees to the chest. Extend the legs back down before landing in a semi-squat position.

Box Jumps

Directly facing the jump box and standing stationary, leap up with both feet and land on the box. Be sure to fully extend the calves for maximum emphasis on the calf muscles.

Lateral Box Jumps

Standing to the side of the box with both feet together, jump sideways (keeping the feet together and bringing the knees to the chest similar to the tuck jumps) clearing the box and landing on the other side. Jump back to the original side and repeat as needed.

Depth Jumps

Standing flat-footed atop a box, bring your arms behind you and at the same time, bend at the knees. As you thrust your arms forward, leap up and away from the box. Focus on getting as much vertical height as possible. Once you land, allow the body to motion downward into a squat position and then jump again, fully extending your body in a vertical fashion (as you would for squat jumps). Remember to land with a slight squatting motion. As a tip, you can set up multiple boxes to repeat the motion quickly.

Squat Throws (Medicine Ball Required)

Stand with feet slightly wider than hip-width apart, and with knees slightly bent. Hold medicine ball at chest level and squat down to a parallel position. Quickly explode up and jump as high as you can. As you start your jump you should start to shoulder press the ball up and reach full extensions with the arms when you are at the peak of your jump. Push ball as high as possible into the air. Try to minimize the time spent in the squatted position. It should be a quick squat and jump. Catch ball on the bounce and repeat according to prescribed repetitions.

Single Arm Overhead Throws (Medicine Ball Required)

Stand with feet slightly wider than hip width apart. Grasp medicine and lower body into a semi-squat position. Explode up extending the entire body and throwing the medicine ball up into the air. The aim is to throw the ball as high as you can and generating most of the power in the legs. Catch ball on the bounce and repeat.

Plyometric Push-Ups

Start by getting into a push-up position. Lower yourself to the ground and then explosively push up so that your hands leave the ground. Catch your fall with your hands and immediately lower yourself into a push-up again and repeat.

Overhead Throws (Medicine Ball Required)

Stand with one foot in front (staggered stance) with knees slightly bent. Pull medicine ball back behind head and forcefully throw ball forward as far as possible into the wall. Catch ball on the bounce from the wall and repeat according to prescribed repetitions. Keep the time between pulling the ball back and starting the throw (transition phase) to a minimum. This can also be completed with a partner instead of a wall.

Side Throws (Medicine Ball Required)

Stand with feet hip-width apart; place left foot approximately one foot in front of right foot. Hold medicine ball with both hands and arms only slightly bent. Swing ball over to the right hip and forcefully underhand toss ball forward to a partner or wall. Keep the stomach drawn in to maximize proper usage of muscle. Catch ball on the bounce from your partner or wall and repeat.

Over Back Toss (Medicine Ball Required)

Stand with feet slightly wider than hip width apart. Have a partner or trainer stand approximately 10-15 yards behind you. Grasp ball and lower body into a semi-squat position. Explode up extending the entire body and throwing medicine ball up and over the body. The goal is to throw the ball behind you as far as you can by generating most of the power from the legs. Catch ball on the bounce from your partner and repeat according to prescribed repetitions.

Ball Slams (Medicine Ball Required)

Stand with feet parallel, shoulder-width apart and knees slightly bent. Pull medicine ball back behind head and forcefully throw ball down on the ground as hard as possible. Catch the ball on the bounce from the ground and repeat according to prescribed repetitions.

Many people combine plyometrics and calisthenics to create workout routines. The use of these two forms of exercising is very popular in **HIIT** and **Tabata** based training. In fact, many people prefer this type of training over going to the gym. **HIIT**, or **high-intensity interval training**, describes any workout that alternates between intense bursts of activity and fixed periods of less-intense activity or even complete rest. It is without question one of the most effective and efficient ways to burn fat and boost aerobic capacity. Here is an example of a **HIIT** workout using Plyometrics and Calisthenics.

HIIT Workout

-Perform 10 Burpees

-Then jog in place slowly for 30 seconds

-Perform 15 Squat Jumps

-Then jog in place slowly for 45 seconds

-Perform 20 Jumping Jacks

-Then jog in place slowly 60 seconds

-Perform 20 Jumping Jacks

-Then jog in place slowly for 60 seconds

-Perform 15 Squat Jumps

-Then jog in place slowly for 45 seconds

-Perform 10 Burpees

-Then jog in place slowly for 30 seconds

Then you could repeat the routine above if you wished to add length to your workout.

Tabata training is High Intensity Interval Training (H.I.I.T) workouts that last four minutes. With Tabata training you work hard for 20 seconds then you rest for 10 seconds. It doesn't seem like it would be that difficult, but that four minutes is the longest four minutes you'll probably ever encounter. Below is an example of a Tabata workout.

TABATA Workout

-Perform Burpees for 20 seconds

-Rest for 10 seconds

-Perform Burpees for 20 seconds

-Rest for 10 seconds

-Perform Squat Jumps 20 seconds

-Rest for 10 seconds

-Perform Squat Jumps 20 seconds

-Rest for 10 seconds

-Perform Jumping Jacks for 20 seconds

-Rest for 10 seconds

-Perform Jumping Jacks for 20 seconds

-Rest for 10 seconds

-Perform Push-ups for 20 seconds

-Rest for 10 seconds

-Perform Push-ups for 20 seconds

-Rest for 10 seconds

This adds up to one four minute round. If you're feeling brave or not challenged, repeat for a second round.

Bottom line you don't need a gym to workout. So if you're feeling light on cash, there's no reason you can't get your sweat on. Not to mention, many gyms offer memberships below twenty dollars a month. That's not even 65 cents a day, so stop using your wallet as an excuse not to exercise.

Let's move on to the cost of eating healthy.

I can't keep track of how many times I've watched people try to justify their poor eating habits by claiming that eating healthy was too expensive. I have no problem admitting that food prices are increasing, especially the price of many nutrient-dense healthy foods. However, here is some advice on how to keep your costs down while also maintaining a healthy diet.

Right off the bat, avoid fast food restaurants as well as food marts a.k.a. convenience stores. I know many of you live very engaged and stressful lives, but you have to realize how much extra you're paying (health-wise and money-wise) for the bullshit food you buy at fast food restaurants and food marts. Here's a back-up plan for when you're pressed for time or in a rush. Instead of spending 5 to 6 dollars on fast food, run into the grocery store and spend 4-5 dollars on a pre-made salad, or maybe 3-4 dollars on an apple, yogurt, and a bottle of water. You can get 2 of those "tuna lunch kits" (tuna, crackers, light mayo and relish) for under three dollars, then add a piece of fruit to round out your meal. If you must patronize a food mart, buy some packaged nuts, a low-fat yogurt drink, or a nutrition bar. Just remember to buy enough to hold you over until you can get home, or somewhere where you can get a decently priced, nutritious meal.

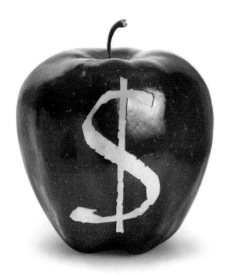

Fruits and vegetables are always part of a healthy diet. It's also one component of a healthy diet that can be expensive if you don't spend your money wisely. Here are some things to remember when buying your fruits and vegetables. First, choose the fruits that are in season. Second, buy your fruits in a bag as opposed to buying them individually. Third, buy frozen fruits and vegetables if you're really tight on cash. Frozen fruits and vegetables are just as nutritious as the fresh ones, plus they're perfect for smoothies. They also can be used as an ice pack to keep the rest of your packed meal cold while they are thawing out.

Buying protein might be the biggest complaint I've heard over the years when it comes to draining your wallet. Still, protein is an important part of a healthy diet and we can't skip out on it. Many people only buy and consume the expensive protein sources like lean meats, fish, and chicken. However, the cheapest sources of protein are canned beans, canned tuna, eggs, milk, and even peanut butter. Including these protein sources in your diet, and using the other sources more sparingly will take your money a lot further.

Start drinking water! Soda's cost money and do absolutely nothing for you, except wreck your diet. Yes, I know bottled water costs money too, but it's still less than diet soda and sugar loaded beverages. Besides you can always drink tap water at no cost. It's just as healthy as bottled water. If you absolutely have to have something besides water, then Crystal Light will not dent your wallet. It costs about one cent per ounce when mixed. All the same, Crystal Light does contain artificial sweeteners and we've already covered what they do to your body.

Remind yourself that a healthy diet consists of a variety of whole grains, fruits, veggies, fish, lean meats, poultry, as well as some low-fat dairy. Understand that even though baked chips, low-fat processed foods, and pretzels are better for your heart and have fewer calories, they still are not essential for a healthy diet. They simply are the lesser of two evils. I know, baked chips may be "better for you" than regular chips. However, I also know that they cost more than regular chips and more importantly are not part of a healthy diet. This also applies to most prepared and pre-packaged snack items, soda, candy and alcohol. If you are really trying to watch your budget, save the 3-4 bucks that you would have spent on a bag of baked chips and spend it on some fresh or frozen produce that is essential! Your outlook on being healthy can control a lot of things, even how you prioritize your spending. Try investing a little more money towards a healthy diet, and a little less on non-essentials like alcohol, fast food, manicures, entertainment equipment, and personal gifts for yourself. Look at it from this perspective, spending money on a healthy diet today may prevent you from having to pay enormous medical bills related to deteriorating health in the near future. Contribute towards a healthy body today because your future health depends on it.

Last, there's the complaint about how much workout clothes cost. This is by far the lamest, off all protests I hear about the cost of fitness.

First of all, only spend money on what you absolutely need. Have a few warm weather outfits, and a few cold weather outfits to get you through the week and between washes. Second, stay away from designer brands, use coupons and buy on clearance. Third, take care of the outfits you buy so they'll last longer. Avoid machine washing everything, and hang dry as an alternative, it will preserve your outfits.

Before we move on to the next chapter, take this quick quiz to see how much you absorbed reading this Chapter on Overcoming Obstacles.

Chapter 4 Quiz

1. **Which of the following is an external obstacle?**

   a) Emergency

   b) Money

   c) Motivation

   d) None of the above

2. **Which of the following is an internal obstacle?**

   a) Time

   b) Being tired

   c) Confidence

   d) All of the above

3. **Which of the following is an example of HIIT Training?**

   a) Running

   b) Calisthenics

   c) Plyometrics

   d) Tabata training

   e) All of the above

4. **Which of the following is a great way to save money while improving your fitness?**

   a) Buy fruits when they're in season

   b) Stay away from designer exercise clothes

   c) Rob a bank

   d) A and B

   e) None of the above

Answers to the quiz can be found in the back of the book

Be grateful for all the obstacles in your life, because they will strengthen you as you continue your journey

Onto Chapter 5

CHAPTER five
LIFESTYLE

When I decided to write this book, I had one thing in mind. Write a book that will not only educate people on how to get in shape, but more importantly a book that will teach them to stay in shape. The sad fact is about half of those who start a new exercise or diet program, abandon it within three to six months. The reasons vary, some say it's taking too long, others complain about being hungry or that they miss their favorite foods. Then there are those that just hate exercising, and let's not forget about the ones that bitch and moan that nothing has worked for them. The first four chapters of this book taught you about Structure, Consistency, Habits (Bad and Good), and Overcoming Obstacles. Combining what you've learned from these earlier chapters will be pertinent in helping you to create and keep up a healthy lifestyle. Remember, you need to know exactly what you're trying to accomplish, you must feel passionate about your goals, and you need a solid realistic plan of action. These are the elements which distinguish your goals from your dreams. Let's cover some methods that can help you in succeeding to obtain your goals and the healthy lifestyle you deserve, despite any obstacles or challenges that may try to derail you.

First, know exactly what your goals are. If you recall earlier in this book I stressed the importance of goals. Once you have your goals set, clarify to yourself exactly what those goals are. What will accomplishing those goals really look like? Envision this thoroughly, dive into it with compassion and have fun. Your success will depend on how clear you are about your goals. If your goal is to look great in a swim suit, what will that look like? Maybe you want to be able to run

10 miles? Do you want your physician to give you two thumbs up at your next physical? Do you want to have more energy to play with your children? How is the goal you're aiming for different from your current lifestyle? One of the best ways in accomplishing a goal and getting what you want is analyzing it in as much detail as possible. This can be hard to do, and sometimes people struggle with it. However, getting that clear mental picture will provide the focus necessary to achieve your goal.

Second, be ready to pay a price. Being successful at anything takes dedicated planning and effort. In the beginning, all you have is an unclear idea. Then you develop an entire set of plans and immediately move closer to success. That's why the chapter in this book on structure is so important. The same is true when creating a healthier lifestyle, or improving your overall fitness. In your planning and goal setting, take into account the price you will be willing to pay. You ask, "What is this "price"? Well improving your fitness might mean a little less time with your children or partner. That's why you might want to create a plan that works them into the equation. For example, working out with your partner, or walking around the track when the kids are at soccer. In addition it might mean less of a social life, or making healthy decisions when participating in social activities, like passing up alcohol every once in a while. If your life is already congested, there is no room for something new. So the "price" will be carving out the time from these other commitments, so you'll have room for exercise and meal preparation. Make sure that's included in your plan.

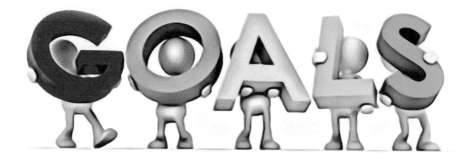

Third, focus on your goal every day. All of us want to achieve our goals as soon as possible, and that's why being focused daily on our goals is very important. This is where the chapter earlier in this book on consistency comes into play. Consistent daily focus is necessary to "burn in" the new neural pathways you need to create your new situation/goal. For example, think of your mind as a piece of clay. The more repeated thought, action or experience, the deeper the groove. All of your previous habits such as eating poorly and not exercising, have etched deep grooves into your mind. Now your subconscious is strong and if you let it, it can fight against you. Likewise, it can be your greatest source of power. Your subconscious thoughts will always try to travel around your brain as quickly as possible using the easiest path, and the easiest path is the one that possesses the deepest grooves. Therefore, the deep grooves only grow deeper as they are travelled along more frequently, and this is the reason people become habitual and are shaped by their thoughts. This is why it is imperative to focus on your goals every day. It's a way of retraining the brain, and carving those deep positive grooves into the mind. The only way to override subconscious anti-success messages is to consciously focus on what you do want, and build new positive neural networks! That is why success is an everyday event. Start out each day committing to your goals, and do not let your goals get buried under the burdens and distractions that will try to take over. Just stay on your new course one day at a time, and focus on your goal and your positive gains.

Fourth, get passionate about your goals. Passion is a strong and intense emotion, and studies have shown that intense emotion is an essential tool to succeeding. Success comes when you do what you are most passionate about! One of the biggest things that most of us lack is passion. Ask any successful person, entrepreneur, millionaire and they will all tell you the same thing… you must be passionate about what you do! So be passionate about bettering your fitness and the goals you've created to get you there.

Finally, take action and consistently do it. Snap out of over thinking and just go do it. There's a reason Nike's slogan is "Just Do it". Jump out of bed in the morning and go exercise, before your brain figures out what's going on dammit. Taking action quickly allows less time for you to create a resistance to eating correctly and exercising. Be accountable to yourself, and if you're working out or dieting with a friend, be accountable to them. You can spend days and weeks contemplating about what may happen if you take action. So instead of letting your mind get lost in "What if" focus on the "How". In a situation focus on how you can do something, how you can solve a problem and/or achieve your goal.

As humans we find excuses, or ways not to do something. We create obstacles, and cripple ourselves. Then we justify what we have done, even though deep down we know we're full of shit. Creating a new lifestyle takes vision, goal planning, commitment, and passion. Furthermore, when we create a new way of life, we have the power to select.

One of the most important things to remember is that you have choices. You make the decisions, and you call the shots. Decide that you want to improve your fitness, and that you want to maintain and live a healthy vibrant life. Then realize, the way you go about it might be different from the way others go about it, and that's fine because this is your life, your health, and you want to create a comfort zone for yourself. Learn from others, ask questions for advice, and read to educate yourself. This will create more options, more solutions, and spawn new avenues that might be more suited for your personality and behavior. Just because someone else is doing something that has brought them results, that doesn't mean that you have to do it that way, especially if it's out of your comfort zone. Find the options that you enjoy doing the most, and this way you can start to find joy in doing them. Realize that you're the only person on this planet that can use your ability, so put it into play. Whether it's creating and modifying workouts that you enjoy doing, or creating or using recipes that you love making…find your comfort zone, and consistency will follow.

Knowing a little about yourself and your personality goes a long way in this game. Learning what type of eater you are, as well as what types of exercise you hate and enjoy will make your continued fitness journey far more possible.

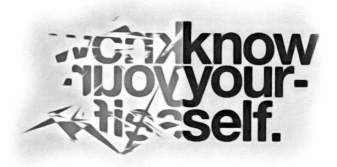

For example when it comes to diet and exercise are you someone who turns to friends or experts for answers. Maybe that's the reason you're reading this book? If this is the case then you're someone that seeks reinforcement, and you might want to consider a weight loss program that meets weekly for fun, companionship, and pointers on nutrition. This doesn't mean that you will have to always use this method, but you do have this choice. Moreover, it could serve as a good way to get you started, get support, and build momentum going forward.

Peer support groups are used in many situations to help people meet their goals, and fitness is no exception. Also consider walking clubs, neighborhood boot camps, or sport-specific clubs or groups. If your fitness routine revolves around a specific activity like dance, cycling, basketball, or martial arts, search for people online in your area who gather routinely. This will give you a regular time and place to take part in the activity. You'll meet new friends who share your passion, expand your fitness network, and probably learn a few things along the way! You could also start your own diet group composed of like-minded dependable friends or associates with interests in weight loss. Also sessions with a personal trainer could give you regular one-on-one help with your specific weight loss obstacles. Another thing to consider is, if you're a big follower that struggles with creating your own methods, choose a diet plan that offers sample meals and grocery lists, similar to one's provided in the first chapter. Plus, surf the internet for workouts and new training methods you can try. YouTube has endless amounts of health, diet, and workout related channels.

How about if you're someone that doesn't like to cook, and you find yourself constantly snacking throughout the day? Maybe your typical snacks consist of bread, peanut butter, chocolate, cookies, cereal, and when you're feeling healthy you reach for yogurt, bananas, or veggies. Whatever the case, when it's time for a real meal that consists of healthy proteins, complex carbohydrates, and good fats...you find yourself to stuffed to polish off that full meal loaded with all the needed nutrients. Then a few hours later you're snacking again on a bunch of bullshit that has no nutritional value. If this sounds like you and you're an obsessive snacker, then choosing a meal plan that requires 4-6 meals a day probably isn't for you, and you might want to consider the following. Strategically place healthy snacks like fruit, nuts, and veggies in places where you're likely to go for them when you need a snack. Meanwhile bury the enemy under the cupboards. Place the cookies, cereals, and potato chips in areas that are inconvenient to reach and out of view. The same applies when at work or on the road, only bring the healthy snacks with you. If you leave the crap behind for healthy choices, then those will be the items you snack on naturally. With this being said, still try to plan for three normal meals that contain predominantly protein. This way you can use your meals to get in your protein, and your snacks as a way to get in some of you complex carbohydrates and healthy fats. Ultimately, you should try to work towards having meals and limiting your snacking, but if you must snack this can help you stay on track. Also consider chewing gum, this helps me from snacking habitually.

Keep in mind that the real goal isn't always finding a diet that works for you. It's finding a way of eating that you appreciate, one which allows you to lose excess weight and keep it off. You may need to reevaluate your diet plan over time as you age and as your lifestyle changes. However, the only way to make it part of your current lifestyle is to find the diet plan that works with you and your personality now.

The same applies towards exercising. Find a way of exercising that you enjoy, you don't have to be at a gym performing cardio and weight training to get in your exercise. These conventional forms of exercise are popular and effective, but a lot of time it's favored by people who are already motivated and not looking for an alternative. Look at your options to improve your fitness, especially if cardio and weight training are not your favorites. Yoga, Pilates, tai chi, and walking, all improve your overall fitness. Many times these alternatives work best for the person who doesn't like high-intensity exercise. These forms of exercise are low intensity, and in most cases don't cause you to sweat a lot. However, they do require movement, burn calories, reduce stress, and are good for people of all ages. Furthermore, research shows that many types of these exercises outperformed aerobic exercise at improving balance, flexibility, pain levels among seniors, and daily energy level.

Workout newbies, the severely obese, the elderly, and people with injuries might find more comfort in functional exercise. It's also great way to get in a workout if you don't have time for the gym one day. Functional fitness programs are designed around exercises and activities that closely mimic the activities of daily living. During the course of the day we change direction, twist, bend, and lift objects at different speeds and in many positions. When we work out on a machine or perform conventional exercises, we do very little to prepare ourselves for the movements of life. In fact, most common injuries occur while performing activities outside of the gym. Functional fitness exercises can increase strength, endurance, flexibility, and balance by using exercises that mimic real life movement patterns. Chopping wood, shoveling snow, cutting the grass, gardening, golfing, walking the dog, cleaning the house, raking leaves, and washing your car are all examples of functional fitness exercise. However, you don't do these activities for 10 minutes and call it quits. You do them for an extended period, like raking leaves for an hour, or taking the dog for a 45 minute walk, and not just around the block to poop. Try gardening for a couple of hours, it's not easy. All of that squatting up and down burns a lot more calories than you think it does. Some other things you can do at home for functional workouts are bodyweight squats, stairs, lunges, push-ups, and planks.

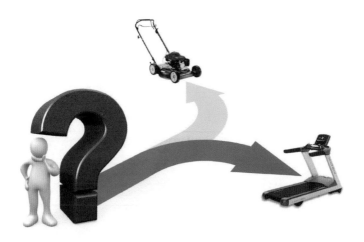

Another option is sports related or recreational exercise. Find a sport that you enjoy doing, or maybe one that you've always had an interest in playing. Sports such as baseball, biking, volleyball, swimming, soccer, skiing, basketball as well as other different games can serve as a very good way to get in exercise. If you enjoy sports and recreation it can serve as an activity that uses physical exertion while also burning loads of calories. Also, you don't need any experience in a sport to fit into this category, just the interest and motivation to learn. Once you figure out what you enjoy the most and what type of exercise personality you own, it'll be easier to exercise, stay consistent, and achieve your goals.

Once you realize you've got choices, the next step is to spend a bit of time with yourself and be selfish. How many times have you thought, "I wish I had a little more time for myself."? Making time for yourself is not something you should feel guilty about. It's nothing more than taking some time to put aside your daily business and treating yourself to something that you want to do. It gives you an opportunity to blow off stress, refocus and recharge. And when you do that, you can come back to your other responsibilities with greater focus, commitment and enjoyment. Many of you have taken care of your loved ones and helped them with the details of their lives they would otherwise miss or overlook. You've been an educator, helper, counselor, and babysitter all wrapped up in one packet. However, who's taking care of you? To care for others, you must care for yourself. As the airplane safety video says, "Put your own oxygen mask on first." because you can't take care of your loved ones if you're running out of oxygen yourself. So don't feel guilty about putting aside time to exercise and improve your health.

When it comes to attaining your fitness goals and improving your health, there will be sacrifices and time restrictions that you will have to place around yourself. Attaining goals comes from being driven internally. I'm sure many of you are still asking, "Is this thinking only of oneself?" The answer is "No". Think of this type of selfishness as investing and protecting. Here's a scenario for you. Let's say you've been consistent with your exercise and diet, you've hit all your goals for the last three months, and you've managed to lose 15 pounds. You're on a roll and nothing is going to derail you. However, your friends are making efforts to thwart your consistent healthy habits. They're mocking you, and claiming that you're obsessive, and saying you're being selfish with your time. Guess what? This means you are taking care of yourself and doing it right! As far as I'm concerned, obsessed is a word the lazy use to describe the dedicated. It also means your friends might be a little envious of your commitment and results.

Finally, embrace your change and new lifestyle. Embracing your changes is important, because change for many is a difficult thing. We aim to control our lives the best we can, but major changes sometimes are overwhelming and in some cases dreadful. However, you must remember one of the beautiful things about life is possessing the ability to re-invent ourselves over and over. It takes bravery, an open mind, and the enthusiasm to take a step towards shaping up, and it takes the ability to laugh it off when you fall down, because eventually you will. Nevertheless, once you get the hang of exercising and eating correctly, the errors and lapses will start to diminish and a sense of pride for your accomplishments sets in.

Don't forget to set reasonable expectations. Unreasonable expectations of life are too often met with loss, disappointment, and pain. Acknowledge that your new lifestyle will be unlike your past one. Acknowledging that there will be changes from day one allows you to make these new revisions to your lifestyle with less resistance. Realize that circumstances will not always turn out the way you want them to, and that's perfectly all right. Embracing an obstacle can help you deal with the change effectively, make the decisive adjustments in your life to embrace the change, and help you move forward after the hurdle. Also grasp that change, and these obstacles can become your most effective teacher, but that's only if you allow yourself to learn from these events. Eventually when you welcome, embrace, and learn from change, you inevitably grow stronger. The ability to continuously accept change and make adjustments in your lifestyle ensures that you'll be able to adhere to a healthy way of life forever. In time, you'll grow stronger, and more confident of your ability. Proactively embracing your new healthy lifestyle will give insight and lessons on how to keep up your desired fitness permanently.

Take this final quick quiz to see how much you absorbed reading this Chapter on Lifestyle.

Chapter 5 Quiz

1. **Which of the following can help you accomplish your goals?**
   a) Knowing exactly what your goals are
   b) Be prepared to pay a price
   c) Stay focused on your goals daily
   d) A and C
   e) A,B, and C

2. **Creating a new lifestyle takes which of the following?**
   a) Vision and goal planning
   b) Commitment and passion
   c) Money
   d) A and B

3. **When creating your healthy lifestyle you should take which of the following into consideration?**
   a) What you enjoy doing
   b) Your personality
   c) Your schedule
   d) All of the above

4. **How would you rate this book**
   a) Informative, mind blowing, and highly motivational
   b) All of the above

Answers to the quiz can be found in the back of the book

Start making the life of your dreams a reality. Change can sometimes be frightening, but it's frightening in a positive and inspiring way. Don't wait for the perfect time, because there really isn't one. People every day decide to have children, and the timing is not always right, but that doesn't prevent them from having their dreams of a family. To many times we trick ourselves into thinking the timing is not right, and the universe is scheming against us. The truth is the universe is not scheming against us, but it's also not going out of its way to maneuver in our favor. Conditions are never perfect and "Someday and tomorrow" are diseases that will take your dreams and goals to the grave with you. Best of luck on your new journey!

Answers to Chapter Quizzes

Chapter 1 Quiz
1) C
2) A
3) B
4) D

Chapter 2 Quiz
1) D
2) A
3) E
4) C

Chapter 3 Quiz
1) A
2) E
3) D
4) A
5) A
6) C
7) E
8) A
9) A
10) D
11) F
12) F

Chapter 4 Quiz
1) A
2) D
3) D
4) D

Chapter 5 Quiz
1) E
2) D
3) D
4) Thanks for purchasing my book.
   I wish you continued success and happiness.

Kevin Daum. "*4 tips for Overcoming Obstacles.*"

http://www.inc.com/kevin-daum/4-tips-for-overcoming-obstacles.html

Gardner, Amanda. "*TV watching raises risk of health problems, dying young.*"

http://www.cnn.com/2011/HEALTH/06/14/tv.watching.unhealthy/

Gibaud, Jonathan. "*3 Ways You Are Being Controlled By Your Mind.*"

http://www.dumblittleman.com/2014/07/3-ways-controlled-mind.html

House, Lauren. "*10 unique diet and exercise motivation tips.*"

http://www.care2.com/greenliving/diet-exercise-motivation-tips.html#ixzz3I9AEja82

Mantell, Dr. Michael. "*When it's okay to be selfish.*"

http://www.acefitness.org/acefit/healthy-living-article/60/4820/when-it-s-okay-to-be-selfish/

Mayo Clinic. "*Nutrition and healthy eating: Don't get sabotaged by added sugar*"

Quinn, Elizabeth. "*Coping with the emotional stress of a sports injury.*"

http://sportsmedicine.about.com/od/sportspsychology/a/Injury_Coping.htm

Ravicz, Dr. Simone. "*Confused About Your Goals? Five critical steps for your success.*"

http://successbraincoach.com/confused-about-your-goals-five-critical-steps-for-your-success/

Wansink, B. & Chandon, P. (2006), *Can low fat nutrition labels lead to obesity?* Journal of

Marketing Research, 43(4), 605-617.

Welsh, J.A. *Journal of the American Medical Association*, April 21, 2010; vol 303: pp 1490-1497.

Zelman, Kathleen M. "*Slow down, you eat too fast.*"

http://www.webmd.com/diet/features/slow-down-you-eat-too-fast

39058650R00065

Made in the USA
Lexington, KY
05 February 2015